HEALTH FOR THE PACIFIC 1

HIV/AIDS and STIs

in Papua New Guinea

Revised Edition

compiled by Jennifer Miller and Andrew Solien

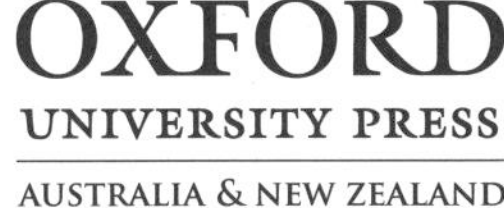
OXFORD
UNIVERSITY PRESS
AUSTRALIA & NEW ZEALAND

Contents

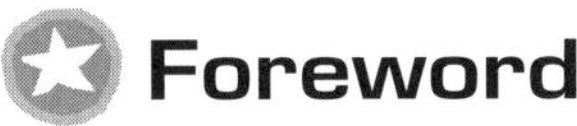

Foreword

The lack of clear, simple and accurate information about good health contributes to poor health in any society.

The Health for the Pacific series is intended to educate and highlight important health issues that are affecting the lives of Papua New Guineans.

HIV and STIs contribute to ill health. Therefore, there is a need to educate our people to be aware of their health, the risks to which they are exposed and the preventive measures that must be taken to avoid infection with HIV and STIs in order to lessen their impact in the communities, villages, towns and cities.

Health is everyone's concern.

I commend the compilers, Andrew Solien and Jennifer Miller, Oxford University Press and the many others who have contributed to the publishing of these health books for schools in Papua New Guinea.

I trust that these books will play an important role in creating a healthy, strong and fit community for a better nation.

Dr Nicholas Mann CMS, MBBS, DCH, FACHSE

Acknowledgments

Papua New Guinea is a rich and diverse culture, with more than 700 languages spoken by its estimated 5.9 million people. It is the biggest island in the South Pacific, apart from Australia (which is also a continent) and Indonesia, with whom it shares its border.

This booklet is a compilation of resource materials written specifically for the education of students throughout Papua New Guinea, and for a variety of people in other institutions. Its aim is to provide education and promote preventative measures that will combat the spread of HIV and the number of people living with AIDS.

I would like to thank and acknowledge the National Department of Health – in particular, Dr Greg Law – for providing technical and other resource materials. I would also like to thank the many people whom I have interviewed while compiling this book. Their time and effort has been invaluable.

Lastly, I would like to thank Oxford University Press for recognising the need to publish health materials for schools in Papua New Guinea.

Andrew Solien

Acknowledgments for the revised edition

Since the original printing of this book by Oxford University Press, significant advances have been made by the PNG National Department of Education towards a coordinated and integrated response to HIV, AIDS and STIs within the primary school curriculum. Amongst these are the HIV/AIDS Policy for the National Education System of Papua New Guinea, the National Department of Education's emphasis on Gender and the HIV&AIDS and Reproductive Health Student Teacher Course Book and Lecturer's Guide.

The second edition of this book, although designed for use by the broader PNG public, complements the PNG Department of Education's primary school subjects Health and Personal Development and is intended as a principal resource for all primary school teachers and students.

I would like to thank and acknowledge the National Department of Education – in particular, Mr Richard Jones – for providing technical and other resource materials.

Lastly, I would like to thank Oxford University Press for recognising the need for a revised edition of this book to address the evolving response to HIV, AIDS and STIs and to support the implementation of Health and Personal Development in primary schools throughout Papua New Guinea.

Jennifer Miller

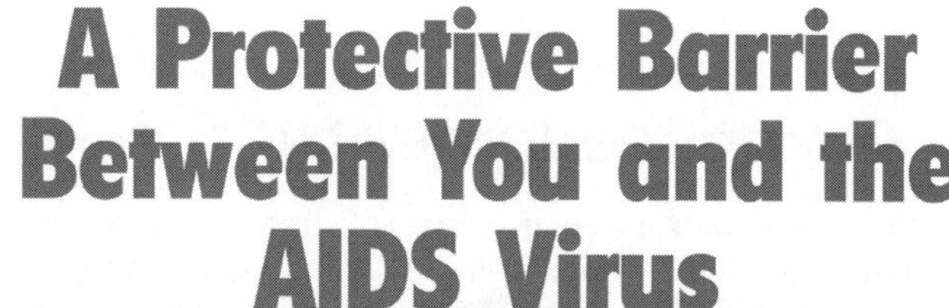

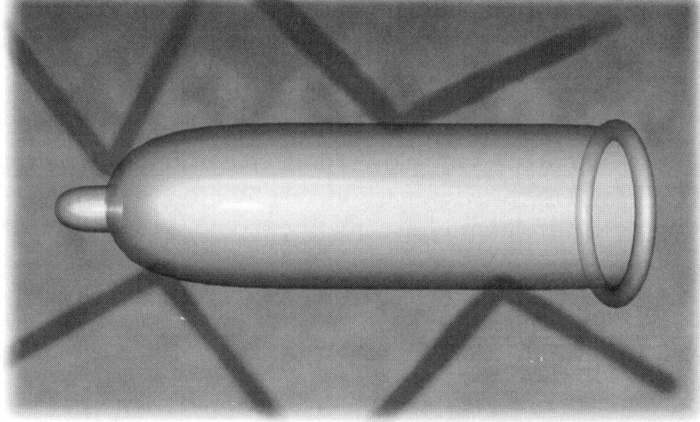

There is no cure for AIDS, and the best ways to protect yourself are not to have sex or be faithful to one partner who is also faithful to you.

But if you do decide to take the risk, you must use a condom *every time you have sex.*

Because, when used correctly, the most effective way to prevent the transmission of the AIDS virus is with a condom.

So, remember...

If you're thinking about sex, think about condoms.

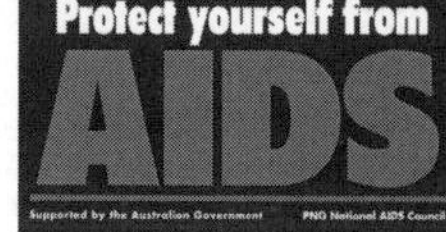

Note to teachers

This student textbook is written for the Papua New Guinea Upper Primary and Lower Secondary subject Personal Development. HIV, AIDS and STIs are some of the most critical subjects in Personal Development. This book supports a life skills teaching approach and contains clear, relevant and accurate information written for Grade 6 and upwards. It has been approved for use in Papua New Guinean schools by the Department of Education and follows the PNG Department of Education HIV/AIDS Policy.

Teachers can use this book in a number of ways: for self study, for the life skills activities, for research in the classroom, and as a resource for other activities. However, a book is not a substitute for interesting, participatory and student-centred teaching and learning. This textbook is designed to complement and support your teaching. Young men and women are at risk of HIV, AIDS and STIs, and schools have a vital part to play in promoting a healthy, responsible lifestyle.

Learning about HIV/AIDS: our schools, our future, our responsibility.

Introduction

The first HIV infection in PNG was reported in 1987. Since then, HIV and AIDS have become serious problems in PNG and the number of reported infections has increased each year. HIV infection has been reported in every district in every province of PNG. In June 2006, the PNG National AIDS Council and the Department of Health reported that 16 104 people had been diagnosed with HIV in PNG. The actual number of people infected with HIV in PNG is far greater than this – approximately 60 000 – because many people do not get tested.

PNG has one of the highest rates of sexually transmitted infections (STIs) in the Pacific. The most common STIs in PNG are gonorrhoea, chlamydia, syphilis, herpes and HIV. Often, STIs do not have signs and symptoms. If left untreated, STIs can cause serious damage to your body and increase your risk of becoming infected with HIV.

HIV, AIDS and STIs are not only a health problem. HIV occurs mostly in sexually active men and women between the ages of 19 and 49 – the age group that is most responsible for social and economic development in PNG. There is no cure for HIV or AIDS. People infected with HIV will have a shortened life and will die. Among those who will die are parents, children, community leaders, teachers, health care workers, politicians, friends and family. However, it is possible to control the spread of HIV and prevent new infections.

There are many reasons why the number of people infected with STIs and HIV continues to increase in PNG – poverty, poor access to education and health services, gender inequality, increased movement within the country, and traditional cultural practices. Information on HIV, AIDS and STIs is often not available or understood by many people living in PNG. The best way to prevent people from becoming infected with STIs and HIV and developing AIDS is to educate them on these subjects. People must learn how to protect themselves, their families and their communities.

This book seeks to provide accurate information on STIs, HIV and AIDS to the people in PNG.

Chapter 1 What are HIV, AIDS and STIs?

HIV stands for Human Immunodeficiency Virus.

H *Human* – This means that the virus lives in and causes disease in people.

I *Immunodeficiency* – This means that the body's immune system is broken down so it can no longer fight diseases.

V *Virus* – This means that this infection is caused by a virus, a very small germ.

AIDS stands for Acquired Immune Deficiency Syndrome.

A *Acquired* – This means that the virus comes from outside your body. To become infected, a person has to do something (or have something done to them) which exposes them to the virus.

I D *Immune Deficiency* – This means that the body's immune system is broken down so it can no longer fight diseases.

S *Syndrome* – This means that AIDS is not one disease. AIDS is a collection of illnesses that a person infected with HIV becomes sick with.

STI stands for Sexually Transmitted Infection.

S *Sexually* – This means that the virus, bacteria or other germ that causes the STI is passed from one person to another through sexual activities.

T *Transmitted* – This means that the infection is passed from one person to another.

I *Infection* – This means that the infection causes an illness in the body.

Questions and Answers

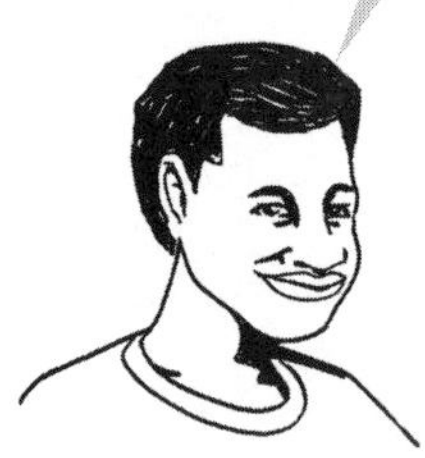

HIV is the virus that causes AIDS. HIV attacks the body's immune system. Most people in PNG who are living with HIV do not know they are infected with the virus and continue to pass it on. People can be infected with HIV for many years and feel healthy. You cannot tell if someone is infected with HIV just by looking at them.

AIDS is the group of diseases that an HIV-infected person becomes sick with. HIV attacks the body's immune system. Over time, the body's immune system is no longer able to defend the body from infections and illnesses. These illnesses are called **opportunistic infections** because they take advantage of the broken immune system. The most common opportunistic infections are tuberculosis (TB), pneumonia and diarrhoea.

HIV is one of the most dangerous STIs, but there are many other STIs in PNG. The number of people infected with STIs is growing each year. Common STIs in PNG include gonorrhoea, chlamydia, syphilis and herpes. Some STIs do not have any symptoms, and people with STIs may not know they are infected. People infected with STIs have a higher risk of becoming infected with and transmitting HIV.

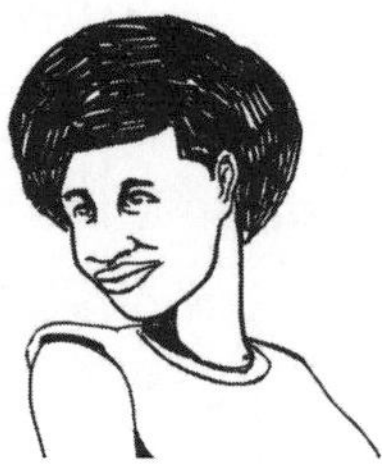

Signs and symptoms of AIDS

AIDS can look very different in different people. Signs and symptoms of AIDS can also look like signs and symptoms of other diseases. The only way to know if you or anybody else is infected with HIV is to have an HIV blood test.

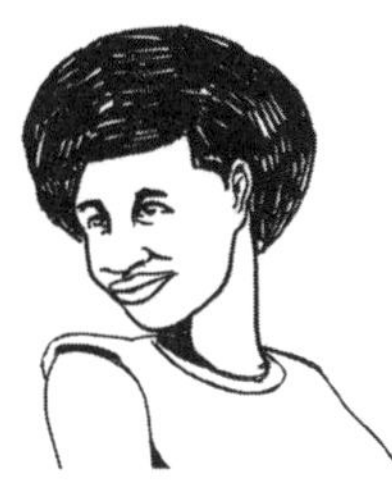
Where did HIV come from?

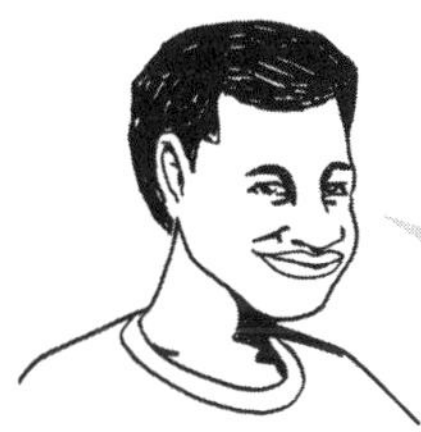
Researchers believe that HIV came from Simian (monkey) Immunodeficiency Virus (SIV) found in chimpanzees in Africa. SIV is very closely related to HIV. In the 1930s SIV crossed to humans when hunters killed chimpanzees that were infected with SIV. The hunters ate infected meat, or blood from the chimpanzee got into the cuts and wounds of the hunters. Once SIV was inside the human body, it quickly changed to HIV. Now HIV spreads from human to human.

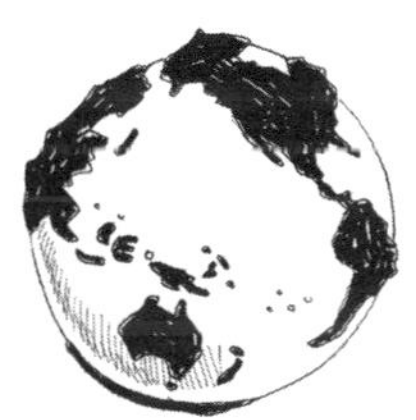

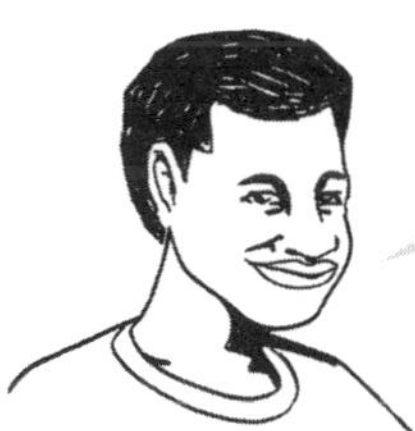
When was HIV first discovered?

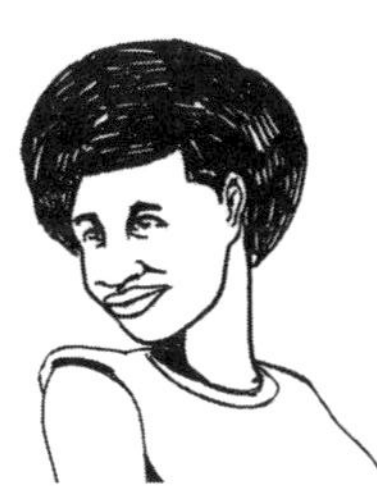
In 1981 the first HIV infection was detected in the USA. Doctors found that healthy men were developing diseases that only happen when the immune system is weakened. These diseases were opportunistic infections. Researchers now believe that in 1981 there were between 100 000 and 300 000 people living with HIV around the world who did not know that they were infected.

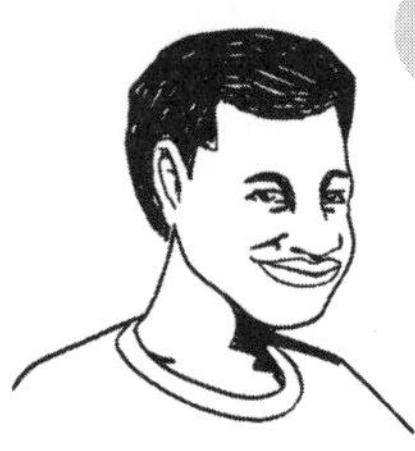
How did HIV spread from Africa to the rest of the world?

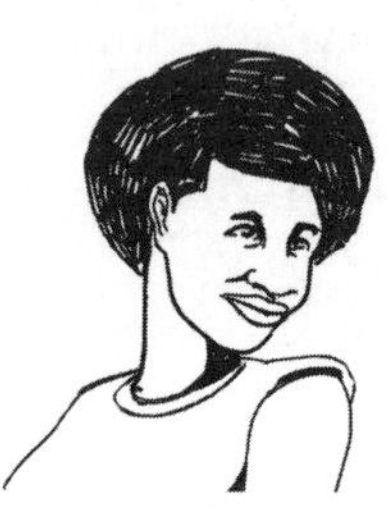
Until the 1980s no one knew about HIV. After the first case of HIV was detected in 1981, the number of cases reported around the world increased very quickly. Researchers believe that travel was the biggest factor that contributed to the spread of HIV around the world.
Throughout the last 100 years, national and international travel has increased in all parts of the world. With many people now travelling on planes, a person living in one city or country can be in a different city or country in the same day.

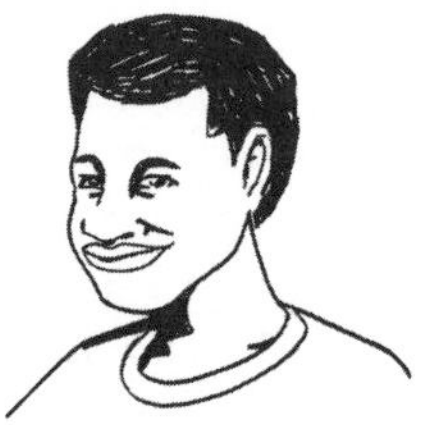
Remember, HIV has no symptoms and AIDS can be mistaken for many other diseases.

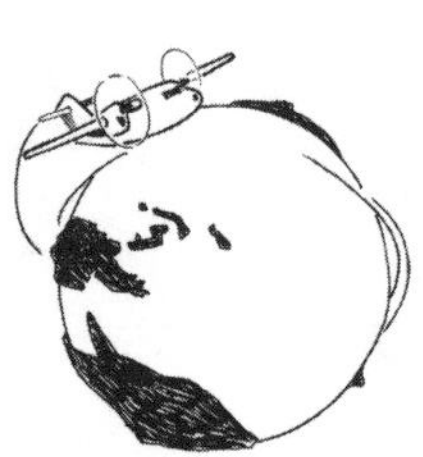

Chapter 2 How does HIV attack your body?

Your immune system

Your immune system works to keep out infections such as:

- **viruses**
  (like flu or HIV)

- **bacteria**
  (like TB or syphilis)

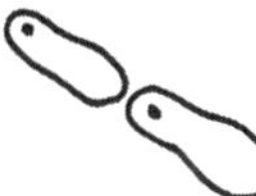

- **parasites**
  (like malaria or worms)

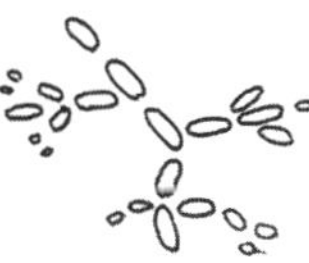

- **fungi**
  (like thrush or ringworm)

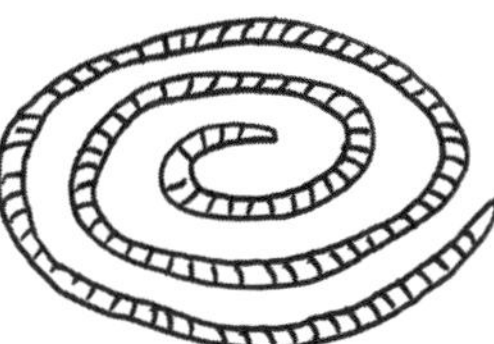

These organisms can infect people and cause disease and death.

Activity 2•1 *Diseases in your community*

Which other diseases do you find in your community?
Sort them into viruses, bacteria, parasites and fungi.

If your immune system meets something from outside the body, such as a virus, it makes small particles called **antibodies**. Antibodies attack viruses and help your immune system to find and destroy the virus, which allows your body to get rid of infections. This helps you avoid illness, or to become well if you are already ill. Your body produces a different antibody for each different kind of infection.

1 Cell releases antibodies

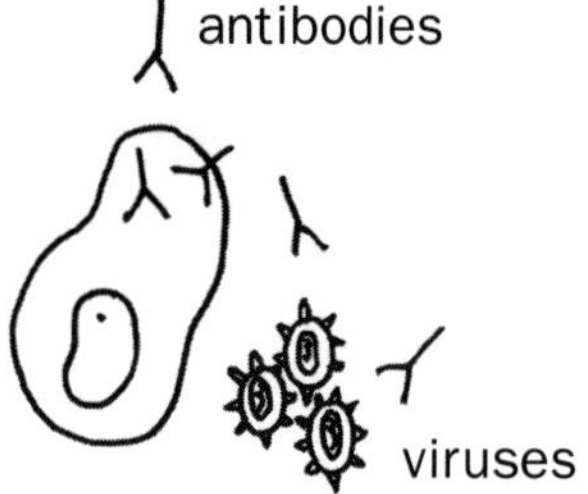

2 Antibodies stick to viruses

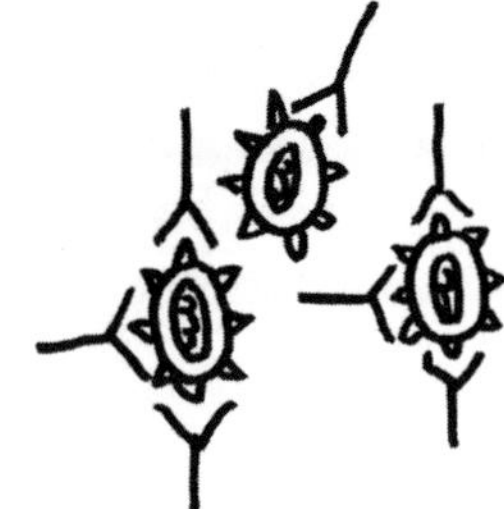

3 Immune system destroys virus

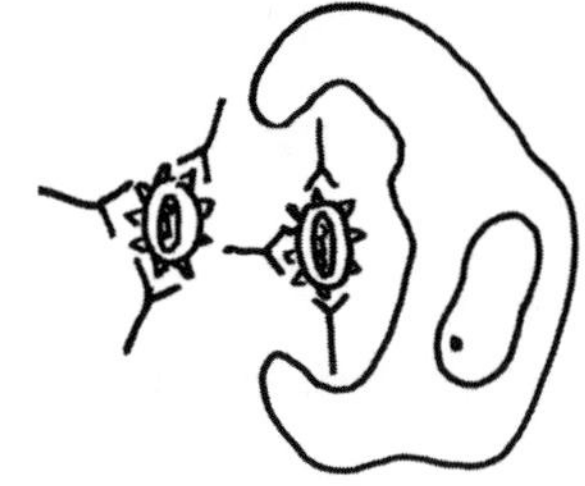

Your body is made up of millions of cells. Cells are tiny parts of a person's body that are too small to see without a microscope. There are many different kinds of cells in your body. Your immune system is made of white blood cells. There are many different kinds of white blood cells, including CD4 T cells.

HIV inside the body

When HIV enters the body:

1. The virus looks for CD4 T cells. These are very important white blood cells.
2. HIV attacks the cell and enters it. The person now has HIV forever. They are HIV-positive.
3. HIV forces the cell to make lots more HIV.
4. The new viruses leave the cell and enter other CD4 T cells and the same thing happens again.
5. Eventually HIV will control many of the body's CD4 T cells. The number of CD4 T cells in the body will go down. This may take many years.
6. The body tries to fight HIV. The immune system creates antibodies against HIV, but these antibodies don't work because HIV is attacking the immune system.
7. Eventually the immune system becomes so weak that the body can no longer defend itself from common illnesses. Bacteria, fungi, viruses and parasites take the 'opportunity' to infect a person with a weak immune system. These illnesses are called **opportunistic** infections. When this starts to happen a person has developed AIDS.
8. People infected with HIV die because their body is not able to defend itself against common diseases like TB, malaria, pneumonia and diarrhoea.

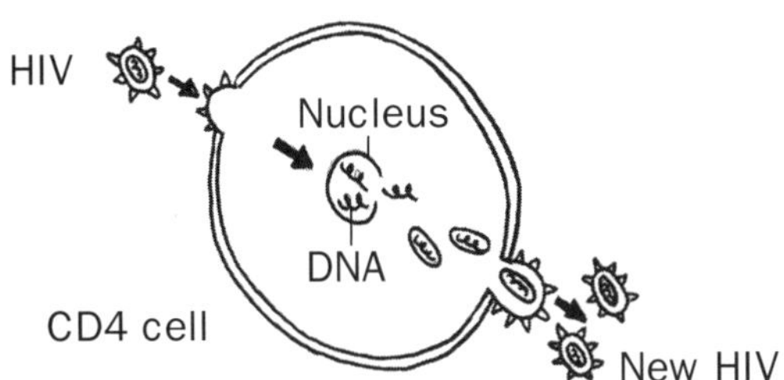

How long does it take for HIV infection to lead to AIDS?

The time it takes for HIV infection to lead to AIDS is different for each person. A lot depends on the health and strength of a person's immune system.

Stress, poor diet and an unhealthy lifestyle and environment can weaken the immune system. In developing countries, such as PNG, a person infected with HIV can generally live between 6–8 years before they get ill and develop AIDS. This might be less or this may be longer. Some people have lived for more than 10 years with HIV and not got sick.

Activity 2·2 *HIV and AIDS Questionnaire*

Conduct a survey in your community about HIV and AIDS. Select five people to interview and ask each person the questions below. Discuss your findings with your parents. Bring your findings back to your school and compare your answers with your classmates. Who knows the most about HIV and AIDS in your community? Why? Your teacher may like to help you by organising a debate about HIV and AIDS.

Age: ______ Sex: ___ Marital status: ______________________

Question 1: What is HIV? ______________________

____

Question 2: What is AIDS? ______________________

____

Question 3: Do HIV and AIDS mean the same thing? ______________________

____

Question 4: How does HIV attack the body? ______________________

____

Question 5: How do you know when a person is infected with HIV?

____

____

Write another question to ask people about HIV and AIDS.

____

____

Chapter 3 HIV around the world and in PNG

The global pandemic

Around the world, millions of people are living with and are affected by HIV.

At the end of 2005:

- almost 40 million people were living with HIV around the world
- more than 4 million new HIV infections were detected in 2005 (this is almost the same number of people that live in PNG)
- almost 3 million people had died as a result of HIV infection.

Some other facts about the HIV epidemic around the world:

- 95% of all HIV infections occur in developing countries
- Africa is the global centre of thc AIDS pandcmic
- sub-Saharan Africa is the region most affected by the HIV pandemic – between 600 and 800 people die **every day** of HIV-related causes in the country of South Africa.

Activity 3•1 *Map Study*

Look at the map on the next page. With a partner, use an atlas to find the countries which are most affected by HIV. List these and then discuss why developing countries have the most infected people.

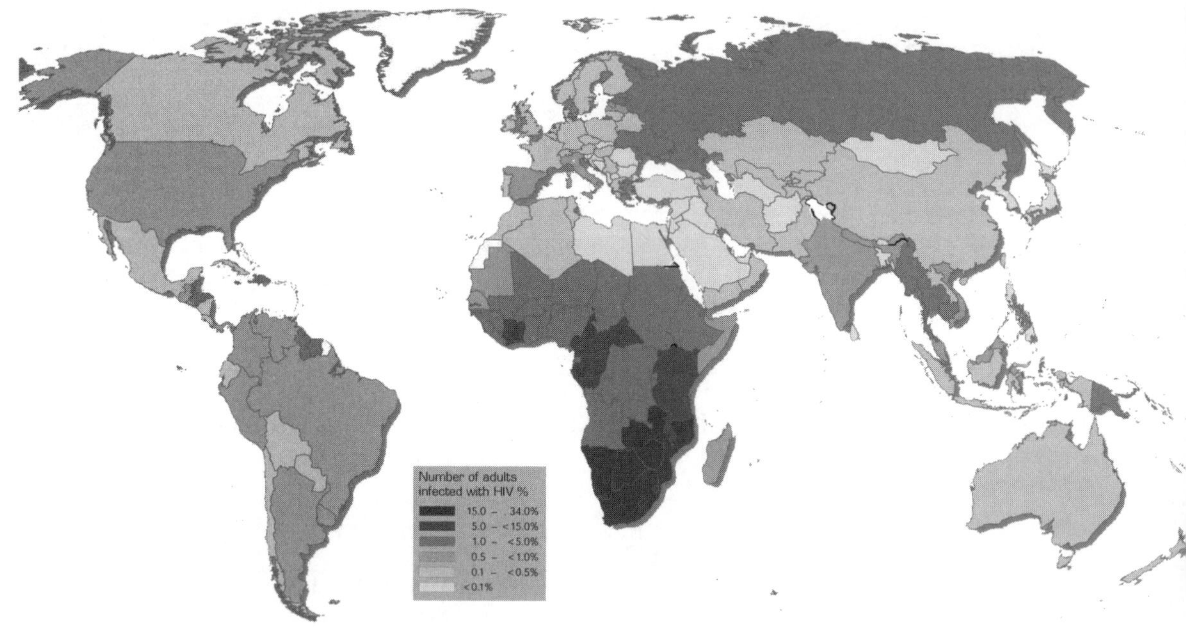

Adapted from A global view of HIV infection: *2006 Global Report prevalence map (pdf). Source: 2006 Report on the global AIDS epidemic, © UNAIDS, May 2006*

HIV in Papua New Guinea

The HIV epidemic in PNG is very serious and is growing very quickly. PNG can learn a lot from other countries that have experienced this epidemic and the terrible effects on their people. Their experiences can help people in PNG prevent HIV and care for those who are already infected and affected by the virus.

- Almost all (90%) of HIV infections reported in the Pacific Region are in PNG.
- More than 1% of adults in PNG are infected with HIV (at least 45 000 people).
- An equal number of men and women are infected.
- Since 1987, the number of HIV infections detected in PNG has increased each year.

HIV infection in PNG, 1987 – 2006

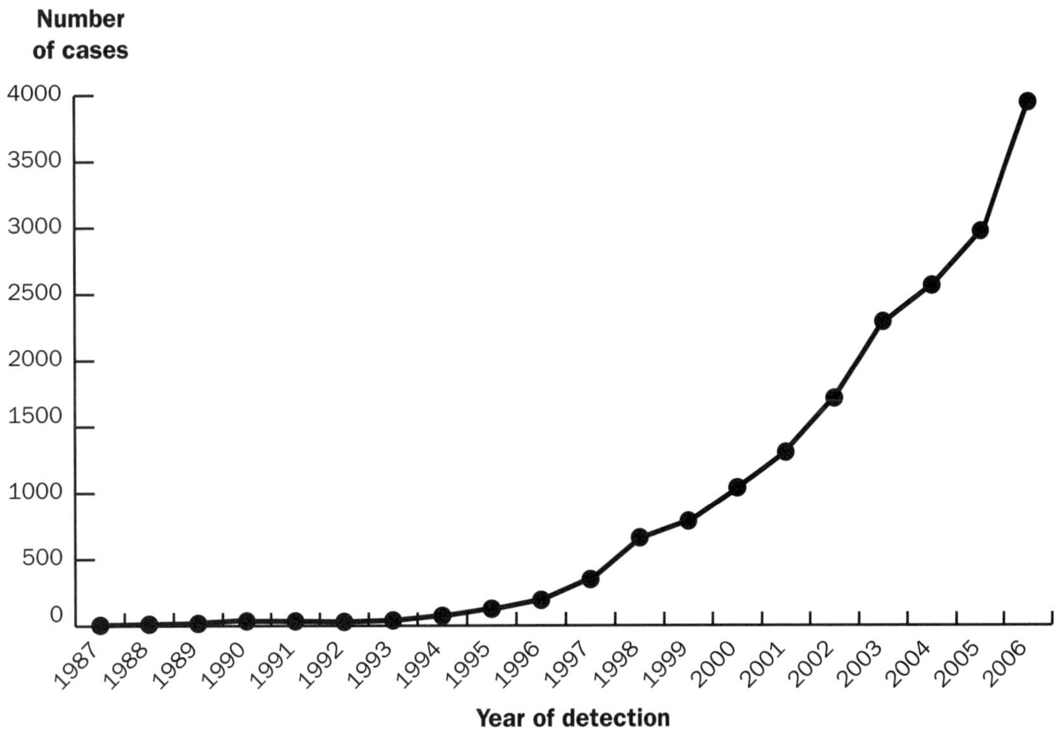

Activity 3·2 *Reading the graph*

The above graph presents the total number of people who became infected with HIV in PNG between 1987 and 2006.

Look at this graph with a friend. What does it tell you?

Remember:

These are only those infections that have been detected with an HIV blood test.

There are thousands of people in PNG who are infected with HIV but do not know this because they have not been tested. Researchers believe that there are actually more than 60 000 people living with HIV in PNG.

HIV infection detected in PNG by age group and sex, 1987 – June 2006

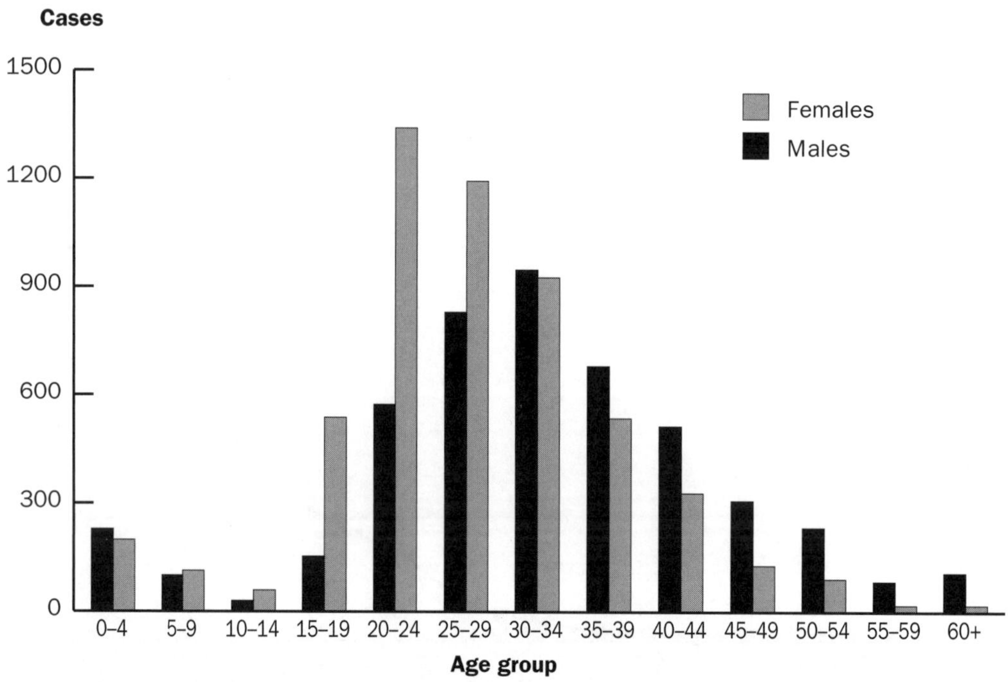

Activity 3·3 *Reading the graph*

The above graph presents the total number of people living with HIV according to whether they are male or female.

With a friend, discuss the graph.

1 What do you notice?

2 Which age groups have lots of HIV infections? Why?

Some interesting information can be learned from the graph:

- Generally, women become infected with HIV at a younger age than men (15 to 34 years of age).
- Generally, men become infected with HIV at an older age than women (25 to 49 years of age).
- These numbers suggest that young women are having sex with older men.

Activity 3·4 *Newspaper Search*

Search the newspapers for stories related to HIV and AIDS. Share and discuss these with your friends.

1 Where else can you find accurate information about HIV and AIDS?

2 Where can you find the latest statistics about HIV and AIDS in PNG?

Why is the HIV epidemic increasing in PNG?

HIV and other STIs are growing problems in PNG. Some reasons for this include:

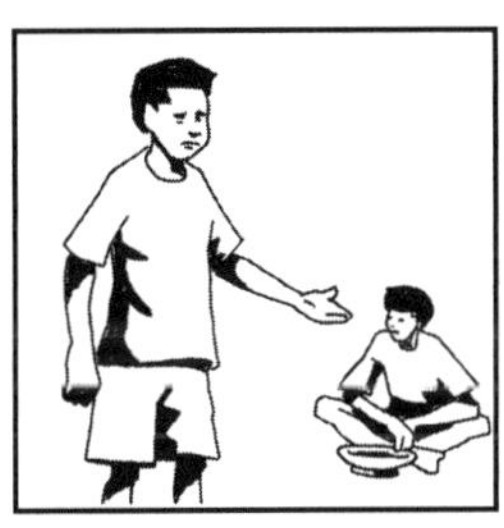

Poverty and unemployment

- These can lead to people having sex in exchange for money and goods as well as other risky sexual behaviours.

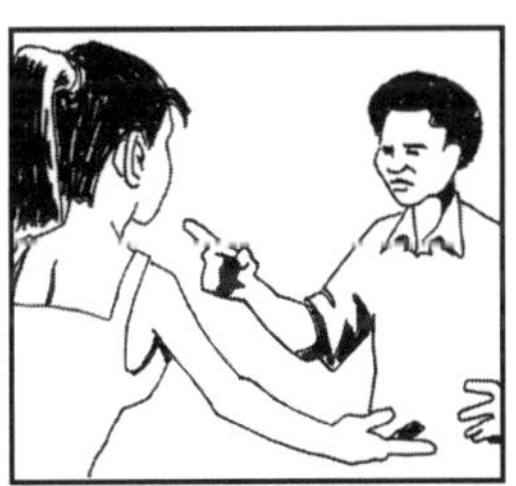

Gender inequality

- Some social and cultural traditions can increase men's power over women. This decreases women's ability to refuse sex or ask to use a condom.

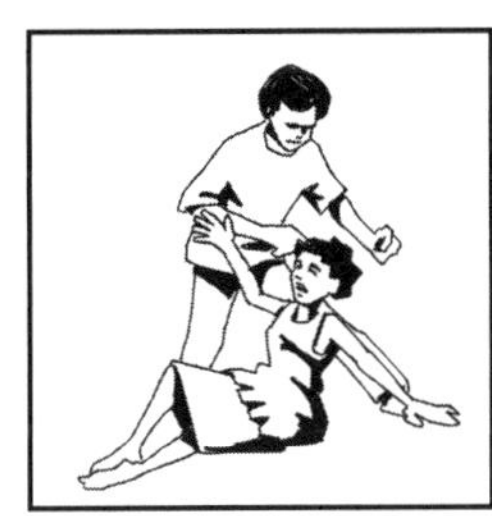

Domestic violence, rape, pack rape and sexual abuse

- Forced sex increases the risk of becoming infected with HIV.

Cultural practices

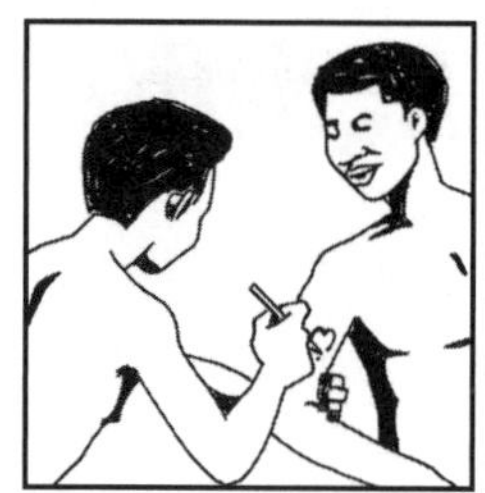

- Tattooing and cutting using unsterilised or shared equipment
- Polygamy

Taboos

- In PNG society, it is often taboo to discuss sex.
- Communities sometimes do not want sex education taught in their schools.

Mobility

- PNG populations are travelling more than ever – from village to town, town to provincial capital, NCD and internationally for work, school and personal reasons.
- People often behave differently when outside of their village and may have different sexual partners or have sex without a condom.

Stigma and discrimination towards people with HIV and AIDS

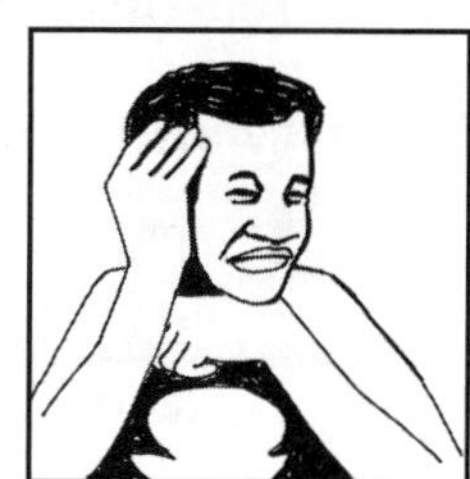

- This makes people scared to get tested for HIV, or to get treatment when they are sick.

High rates of STIs and teenage pregnancies

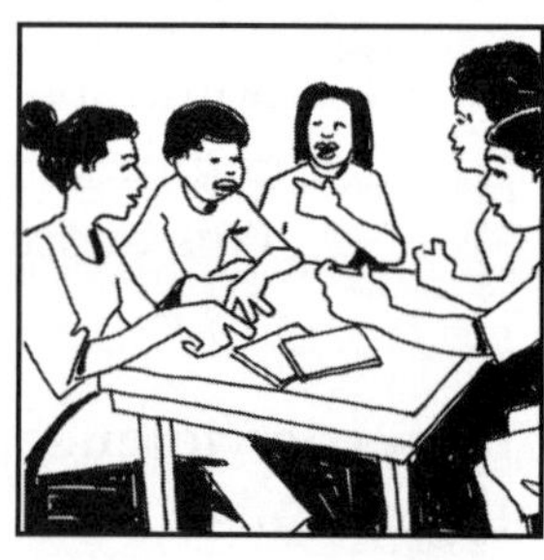

- This shows that many people are having unprotected sex with multiple partners.
- This also shows that young people are having unprotected sex.

Low condom use and opposition to condoms

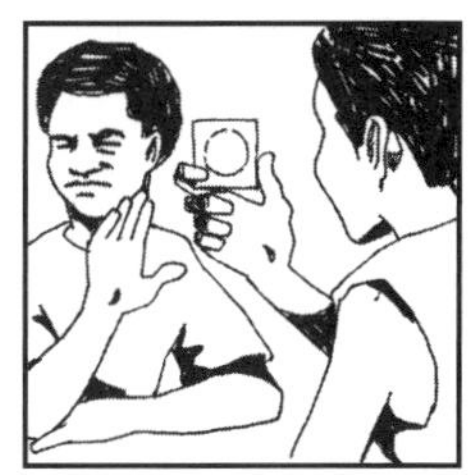

- This means that people don't protect themselves and others.

Alcohol and drug use

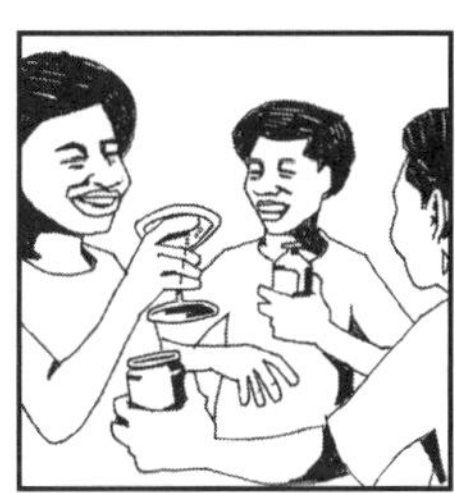

- This can lead to risk-taking and poor decision-making.

Activity 3•4 *My community and HIV*

Think about the above factors that contribute to the HIV epidemic and answer the following questions.

1 Which of these factors exist in your community?
2 What other factors contribute to the spread of HIV in your community?
3 What do you think will happen to your community in the future if we don't stop the epidemic? Discuss your thoughts with your friends and classmates.

CASE STUDY

Jane's story

(This is a true story, but the names have been changed.)

Jane was diagnosed five years ago as being infected with HIV. The doctor told Jane that the HIV virus will stay in her body forever, make her very sick, and eventually kill her. Jane was told that there is no cure for HIV and AIDS. There are some medicines that slow down the effects of HIV, but medicines cannot eliminate the virus completely.

Jane is still strong and healthy, eats nutritious food, and works in her garden. In the beginning, Jane's family and community were scared and sent her away, and Jane was very sad. After some time, Jane's family learned about HIV and invited her back to the community. Now Jane has an understanding family who treat her well.

Jane tries to deal with her illness. She has two children to care for and wants to be able to care for them for many more years.

Jane's husband was a PMV driver. Jane was always faithful to her husband, and believed that he was faithful to her. Jane has learned a lot about HIV and knows that it can be spread through unprotected sex.

Jane thinks about the many times when her husband was working away from the community with his PMV. Jane's husband died two years ago from AIDS-related illnesses. Jane wonders about her husband's sexual activities when he was away. Was he unfaithful? Jane knows that she became infected with HIV from her husband, but she does not know how he became infected.

After reading Jane's story, answer the following questions:

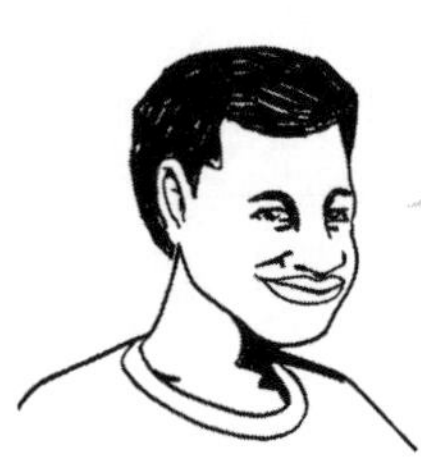

1. How did Jane become infected with HIV?
2. How do you think Jane's husband became infected with HIV?
3. Why do you think Jane's family changed their minds about her?
4. How does Jane keep herself healthy?
5. What lessons can you learn from her story?

Chapter 4 How is HIV spread?

HIV is passed only through blood, semen, vaginal fluids and breast milk. When these fluids enter someone's body, they can be infected with HIV.

There are three main ways of becoming infected with HIV:

Sex – Having sex without a condom with someone who is HIV-infected.

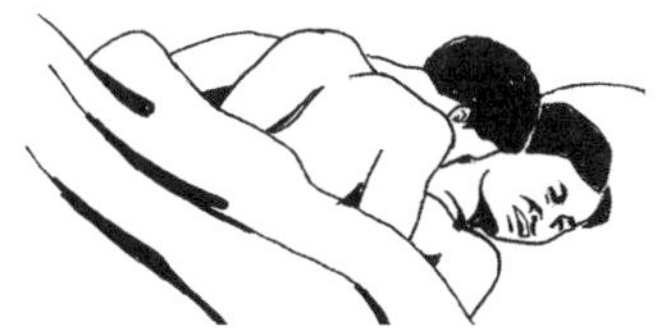

This is the most common way that HIV is transmitted in PNG. HIV can be transmitted through anal and vaginal intercourse. It is very rarely transmitted through oral sex.

Parent to child transmission (PTCT) – An HIV-infected mother can pass the virus to her child during pregnancy, labour and delivery and through breastfeeding. There is a 1-in-3 chance that an HIV-infected mother will pass HIV to her child.

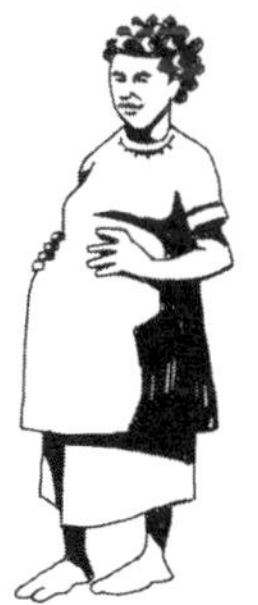

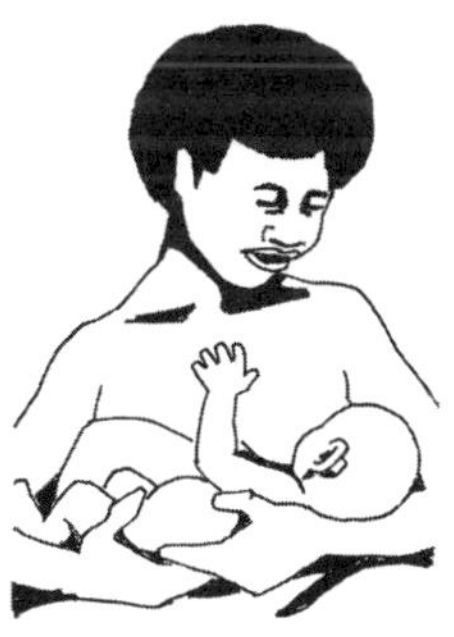

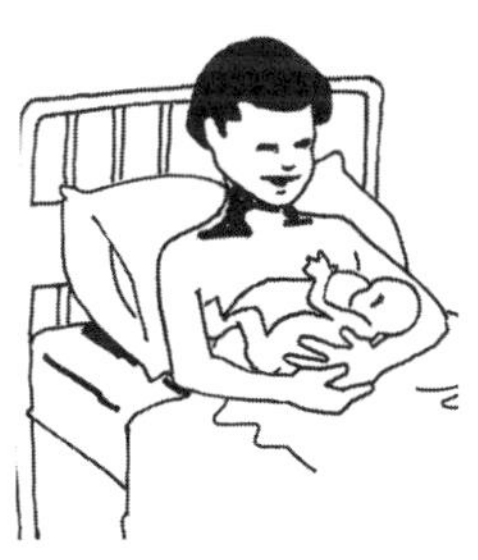

Contact with infected blood – This can occur through sharing of sharp instruments such as needles, razor blades and other skin-cutting instruments.

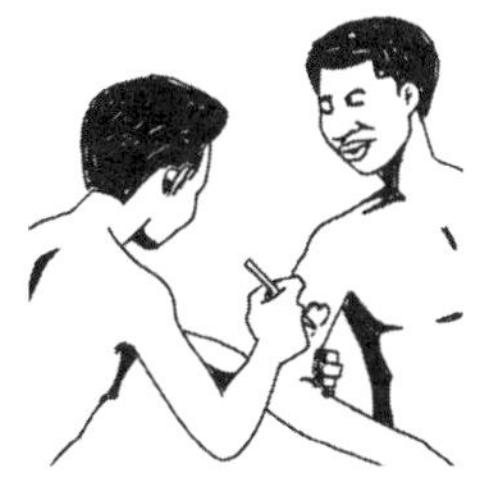

In PNG, blood used for transfusions is tested for HIV, so HIV is not transmitted through blood transfusions.

Injecting drug use is not common in PNG, but where it does happen, sharing needles can transmit HIV.

Tattooing, circumcision and other cutting of the skin are common practices in PNG. Sharing razor blades and other cutting instruments can lead to transmission of HIV.

Is it safe for me to be around someone who is infected with HIV?

It is safe to work, study, play, and live with people infected with HIV. It is also safe for children to be in school with children who are infected with HIV. HIV is only transmitted through semen, blood, vaginal fluids, and breast milk. Other body fluids like saliva, sweat, tears, urine (pee), faeces (poo) or vomit do not transmit HIV. In our daily lives, such exchange of fluid or 'blood-to-blood' contact with others is unusual – even in cases of biting, scratching, accidents or fights.

You **cannot** get infected with HIV by:

- taking care of people living with or affected by HIV and AIDS
- shaking hands
- coughing and sneezing

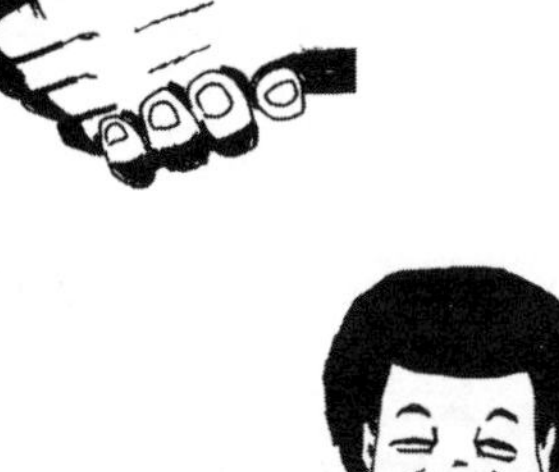

- touching the sweat of an infected person
- sharing food or drinks
- sharing cups, plates, spoons and other eating utensils
- swimming in a pool, river or ocean
- wearing second-hand clothing
- sharing toys

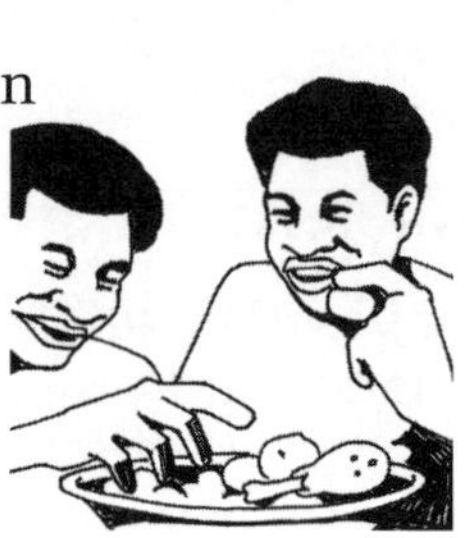

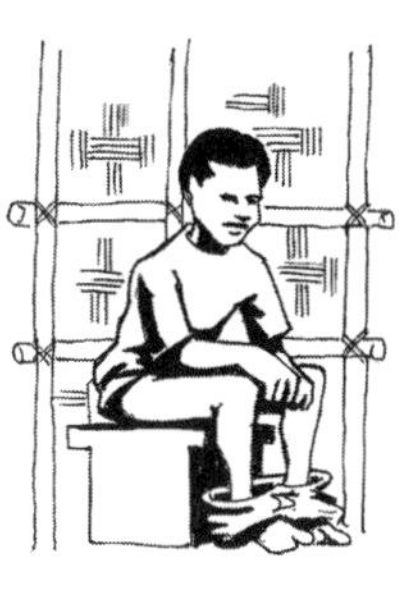

- sharing toilets
- changing nappies
- using PMVs or telephones
- hugging and kissing
- giving blood or getting blood transfusions
- mosquitoes and other insects or animals
- sharing buai or cigarettes.

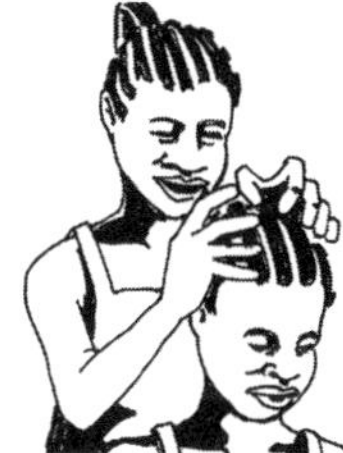

Who can get HIV?

Anyone who has unprotected sex is at risk of becoming infected with HIV.

Anyone who shares sharp skin-cutting or piercing instruments is at risk of becoming infected with HIV.

People are not protected from HIV because they are young, old, a woman, a man or living in a rural area.

People get infected with HIV because of their behaviours that put them or their partner at risk.

Why are men at risk of becoming infected with HIV?

- men tend to have more sexual partners
- young men feel peer pressure to have lots of sexual partners
- cultural pressures and expectations for men to be the 'leader' in sex
- men have more power over women and control sexual activities
- men have more power to decide to use a condom
- traditional practices such as polygamy
- drinking
- travel.

Why are women at risk of becoming infected with HIV?

- HIV is more easily transmitted from men to women because of the larger skin surface of the woman's vagina. There is a bigger chance of women getting small tears during sexual activity
- sexual abuse, rape and forced sex increase the chance of bleeding in the vagina or anus
- there is more HIV present in semen than in vaginal fluids
- poverty puts women at risk. Many women have to exchange sex for money so that they can care for themselves and their children
- although female condoms are available in PNG, women do not often use them
- women have less power than men in PNG culture and cannot control what happens during sexual activities
- unfaithful partners
- many women who refuse sex or request condom use put themselves at risk of being abused or suspected of being unfaithful.

Activity 4.1 *Men's and women's risk factors for becoming infected with HIV*

Think about the above factors that contribute to men's and women's risk for becoming infected with HIV, and answer the following questions.

1. Which of these exist in your community?
2. What other factors contribute to men's risk for becoming infected with HIV?
3. What other factors contribute to women's risk for becoming infected with HIV?
4. Which factors do you think are the most dangerous in your community?

Men and women can reduce their risk of becoming infected with HIV by:

- always carrying and using condoms
- talking about safer sex with their partner(s) before they start sexual activities
- getting tested if they think they have been at risk of becoming infected with HIV – an HIV blood test is the only way to know for sure
- marrying wisely and working with their partner on a strong, faithful and loving marriage.

Activity 4·2 *Protecting yourself from HIV infection*

What other ways can men and women protect themselves from becoming infected with HIV?

Discuss these with your friends and family.

Activity 4·3 *Dilemmas*

Consider the situations below and answer the questions that follow.

1 Your cousin Tom is infected with HIV and you have decided to visit him. When you arrive at his house he is very happy to see you. He comes forward to greet you. What is your response?

2 Your best friend Betty is sick and some of your friends have told you that she is infected with HIV, but you don't believe them. The next day Betty arrives at your house during dinner and you invite her to eat with you. Suddenly, you remember what you have been told about HIV and AIDS. You are worried about what your friends said about Betty being infected. How would you deal with the situation?

3 Work with a friend and write another dilemma and what to do in that situation.

Chapter 5 How to prevent the spread of HIV and STIs

The most common way people become infected with HIV is through unprotected sex. Many people in PNG have unprotected sex without thinking about how dangerous their actions can be. Unprotected sex may result in transmission of HIV and other STIs.

The ABC strategy

The ABC strategy is a national strategy used to prevent the spread of HIV and STIs and to promote safe sex and healthy living. ABC stands for:

Abstinence – This means that a person chooses not to have any kind of sex that could expose them to HIV (no vaginal, anal or oral sex). For young people, this means delaying your first sexual experience. For married people, this means abstaining from sex when you are away from your partner. Abstinence is the surest way to prevent becoming infected with HIV.

Be Faithful – This means that both partners only have sex with each other. Couples must be tested for HIV at a local hospital or clinic.

Condoms – For people having sex, condoms are the only way to protect themselves from becoming infected with HIV. Condoms should be used every time a person has sex to reduce the risk of becoming infected with HIV.

We should all use A and B and C.

Many people in PNG, particularly women, do not have the power or control to follow the ABC strategy.

- Often, women are forced to engage in sexual activities and are not able to abstain.
- Being faithful requires that both partners are faithful to one another. Often one partner may be faithful, but does not know whether their husband or wife is faithful to them.
- Often people do not discuss using a condom with their partner, because they are scared of how their partner will react.

CASE STUDY

Elly and Samson's story

Elly and Samson have been good friends for two years. Samson wants to have sex with Elly and has promised to marry her. Elly and Samson have already had sex once. Elly has heard of HIV and STIs, and does not want to have sex again until she is older. Elly speaks with her best friend Mary about her problem. Mary tells her that no one has to have sex if they don't want to, and nobody should ever be forced into having sex. Mary also says that if Samson really loved Elly, he would respect her feelings and not force her into having sex with him.

The next day Samson and Elly go for a walk and have the following conversation:

Samson: Elly, why don't you want to have sex with me?

Elly: It is not only with you. I just don't want to have sex now.

Samson: We already had sex before. Why are you changing now?

Elly: It would be better for both of us to be safe. We don't want to catch a disease or get pregnant.

Samson: You think I have HIV or another STI? I can't believe it!

Elly: I don't think you have HIV or another STI. But we could both have an infection and not know about it.

Samson: You are being ridiculous. You walked here with me, so you must want to have sex.

Elly: I already said no. I do not want to have sex with you or anyone else right now. Please respect me and my feelings.

After reading Elly and Samson's story, answer the following questions:

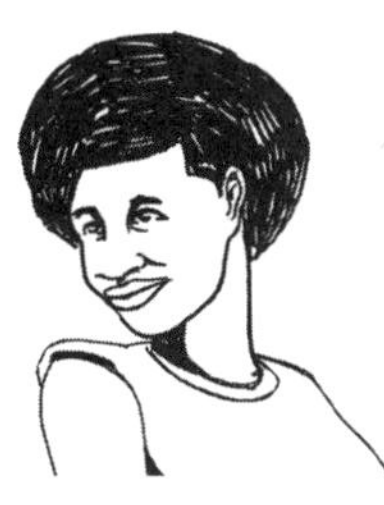

1. What do you think about Samson and what he says?
2. What do you think about Elly and what she says?
3. Is Mary correct in what she said to Elly?
4. What would you do if you were in Samson or Elly's position?
5. Write the next few lines of the conversation between Samson and Elly. Perform their conversation as a role-play.

How to say 'no'

Young people often feel pressured to have sex by their partner or by their friends. It is important for you to have the skills to say no.

You have the right to say 'no' to sex.

The following table presents some examples of different ways young people can say 'no' to sex.

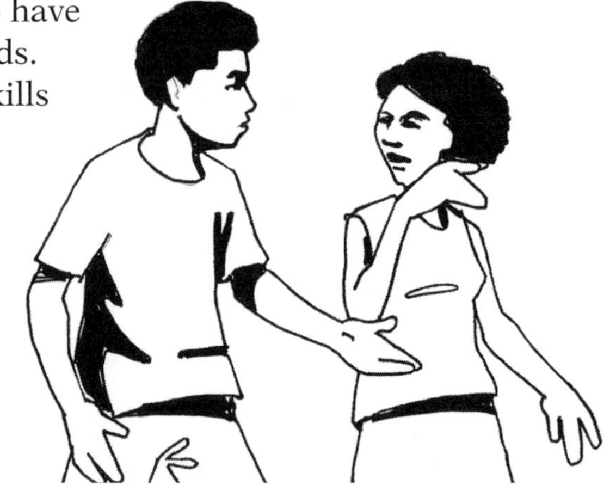

The pressure: Your boyfriend/girlfriend wants to have sex with you.

What you could say to resist this	What they might say to persuade you	What you would say or do if they said this
'No! Even though I like you, I don't want to have sex before I am married.'	'Well, don't worry, because I love you and I will marry you next year.'	'No, if you loved me you would respect my views. Think about it. I will see you tomorrow.'

Activity 5•1 *Saying 'no' to sex*

Work with a friend and list other responses you could say to resist pressure to have sex.

List other ways that people might persuade you to have sex.

Don't forget to say 'no'!

Saying 'no' to sex can be difficult. By resisting pressure and having strong reasons for saying 'no' you can protect yourself from becoming infected with HIV and STIs.

The best ways to resist pressure are:

- say 'no'
- talk about the risks
- talk about your values
- be clear and strong.

Strong reasons for saying 'no' to sex include:

- your parents
- keeping safe from HIV and STIs
- not getting pregnant
- school
- respecting your body
- church values
- feeling under pressure
- what you feel about the other person.

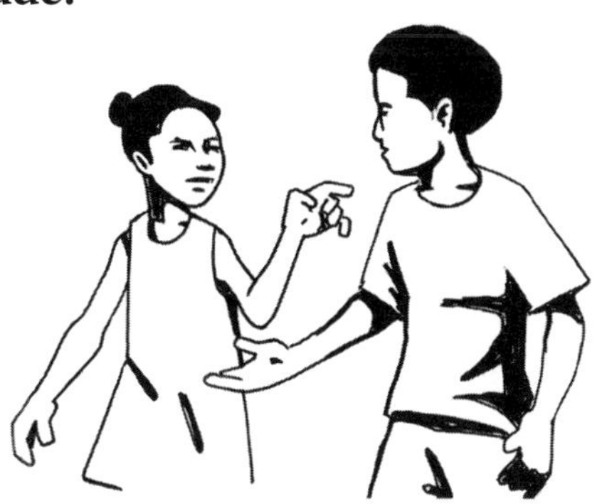

Activity 4.1 *Resisting pressure*

Use the information above to prepare dramas about the following situations:

1. A young couple in which the boyfriend wants to have sex with his girlfriend and the girlfriend doesn't want to have sex.
2. A young couple in which the girlfriend wants to have sex with her boyfriend and the boyfriend doesn't want to have sex.

How can I protect myself and others from HIV infection?

- Don't have sex when you are too young.
- Use condoms every time you have sex.
- Learn as much as you can about HIV and other STIs.
- Marry wisely and work on a strong, faithful and loving marriage.
- When you have symptoms that could be related to HIV and other STIs, visit a doctor or health care worker.
- Have an HIV blood test.

Safe sexual activities

There are many ways of showing affection for another person without having sex. The following are some examples of safer sex, and the level of risk that certain activities have for transmission of HIV and STIs.

Sexual activities that have no risk for transmission of HIV and STIs

- abstaining from sex
- kissing, including 'deep' or open-mouth kissing
- hugging, massaging, touching, rubbing
- masturbating alone or with your partner (rubbing or stroking the penis or clitoris and vagina).

Sexual activities that are low risk for transmission of HIV and STIs

- oral sex (sucking or licking the penis, vagina or clitoris) is considered 'low risk' because saliva doesn't transmit HIV. If you have any fresh cuts or sores in your mouth (even unnoticeable), infected semen, vaginal fluids or blood can enter your bloodstream when you lick or suck a penis, vagina or anus.
- sex with a condom.

Sexual activities that are higher risk for transmission of HIV and STIs

The linings of the vagina and anus are delicate and thin, and can tear easily. These small tears can be invisible and unnoticeable, but enough to let HIV into your body. Therefore the riskiest sexual activities are:

- having vaginal or anal sex without a condom
- having sex too young
- drinking and using drugs, which can lead to people taking risks
- having multiple sexual partners
- polygamy
- rape/gang rape.

Sexual violence and HIV and STIs

Forced sex – rape – increases the risk of becoming infected with HIV and other STIs. This can happen within a relationship or outside a relationship.

People who experience rape (anal or vaginal) are at higher risk of becoming infected with HIV and STIs than would be the case if sex were not forced.

During violent sexual activities, anal and vaginal tissues are easily damaged, which allows HIV and STIs an easier entry into the body.

If you or someone you know is being physically or sexually abused, seek assistance from someone you trust in your community. This person may be a teacher, doctor, police officer or parent.

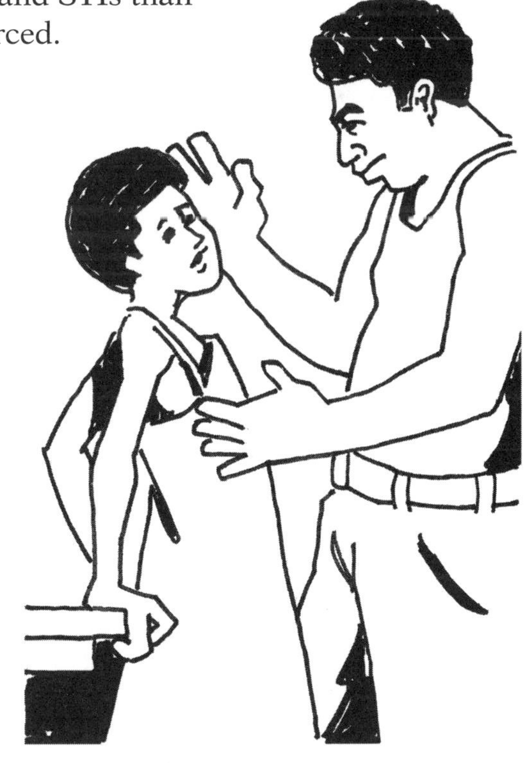

Condoms

Condoms are proven to be an effective barrier against the transmission of HIV and STIs. Using a condom will reduce the risk of infection with HIV or STIs. They are the best protection for men and women who are sexually active if used correctly and consistently. Condoms have stopped millions of men and women around the world from becoming infected with HIV and STIs. Condoms are also a good way to prevent unplanned pregnancy.

In PNG, there are condoms for both men and women – the male condom and the female condom. Condoms are free:

- at hospitals and health centres
- at provincial AIDS committees
- from dispensers in nightclubs, hotels and many workplaces.

Condoms should be stored in a cool dry place. High temperatures, sun and body heat weaken condoms, so don't store them in your wallet or bilum for a long time.

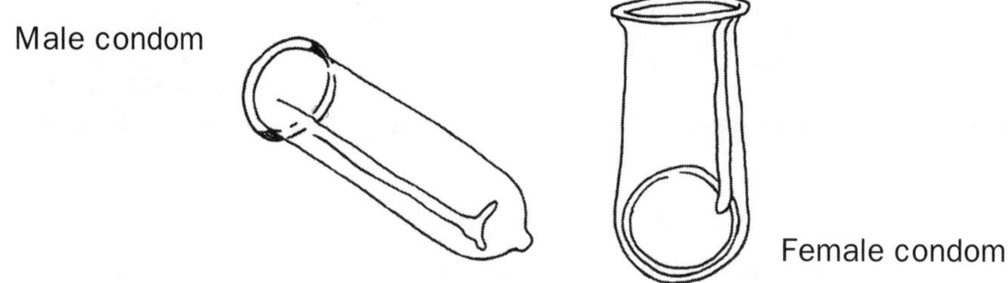

Before you decide to have sex with or without a condom, you should ask yourself and your partner the following questions:

- Do you really want to have sex?
- Does your partner really want to have sex?
- Is either of you feeling under pressure or feeling uncomfortable?

Remember:

- Abstinence is 100% safe.
- Alternatives to sex include masturbation, massaging, rubbing, kissing and hugging.

How to use a female condom

1. Check the wrapper of the female condom. If it is torn or damaged in any way the condom will also be damaged, so throw it away and get another condom. Check the date on the condom wrapper. If the condom has expired, throw it away and use a different condom.
2. Open the condom package carefully. Don't use sharp objects like scissors to open the wrapper. Take care that the condom is not damaged with fingernails, jewellery etc. **You only need to use one condom. Do not use two (e.g. a male and female condom together) – this is risky.**
3. Do not put the erect penis near the vagina until the condom is inside the vagina.
4. Fold the smaller rubber ring (which is inside the condom) into a figure of eight.
5. Insert the ring and the condom deep up inside the vagina so the inner ring springs open near the cervix and holds the condom in place. To make it easier, some women put one leg on a chair or bed to open the vagina further or they lie on their backs with their knees raised.
6. The outer, larger ring should be outside the vagina. Putting lubricant inside the condom makes sex better and safer.
7. The man can now enter the woman, they can have sex and he can ejaculate safely – the condom acts as a barrier to the semen and vaginal fluid.
8. Remove the condom carefully by twisting it, tie it in a knot, and throw it in a pit latrine or bury or burn it. Do not flush it down a Western toilet!

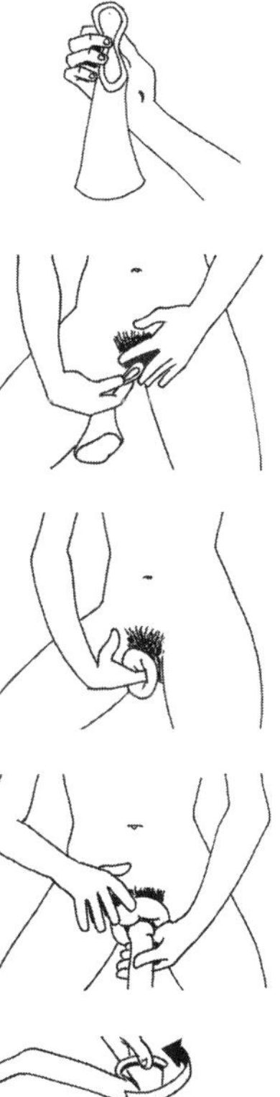

Women need to practise putting in the female condom so if they want to use it they can use it correctly and confidently.

How to use a male condom

1. Check the wrapper of your condom. If it is torn or damaged in any way the condom will also be damaged, so throw it away and get another condom. Check the date on the condom. If the condom has expired, throw it away and use a different condom.

2. Open the condom package carefully. Don't use sharp objects like scissors to open the wrapper. Take care that the condom is not damaged by fingernails, jewellery etc. **You only need to use one condom. Do not use two.**

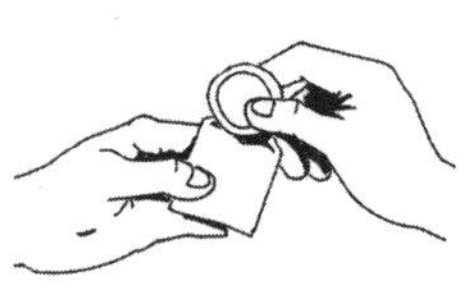

3. Make sure the condom is the right way around. Press out the air at the tip of the condom before putting it on – an air bubble in the condom could result in the condom tearing or falling off. Make sure the foreskin is pulled back before you put on the condom.

4. With the rolled rim on the outside, put the condom over the erect penis. Unroll the condom down over the entire erect penis. Be careful to put the condom on before there is contact with your partner's vaginal area.

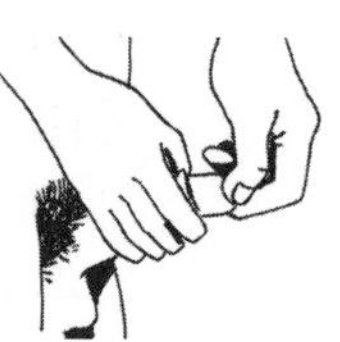

5. Smooth out any air bubbles and check that the condom fits securely. You can spread water-based lubricant on the outside of the condom. It will help reduce friction during sex. **Never** use oil or Vaseline – they damage the condom.

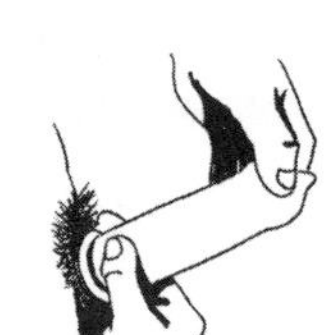

6. After ejaculation, but before the penis is soft, hold the condom firmly at the rim and carefully withdraw from your partner. This is to ensure that semen does not leak.

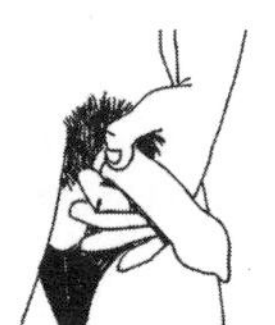

7. **Only use a condom once.** Tie it up and throw the condom and the packet away into a pit toilet or rubbish bin or bury it. **Do not** flush it down a toilet – you will block the toilet!

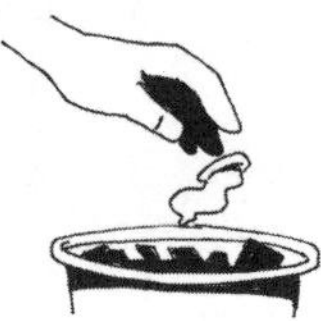

Men need to practise putting on a condom so they will be able to use them correctly and confidently if they have sex.

CASE STUDY

Elisabeth and Mathias

Elisabeth and Mathias are walking down a deserted road in the late evening. Mathias suggests that they walk down a small path and Elisabeth agrees. When they get to an open area, Mathias begins to pressure Elisabeth to have sex with him. Elisabeth tells Mathias that she will have sex with him, but only if they use a condom. Elisabeth has heard of HIV and STIs and wants to protect herself. Mathias does not want to use a condom.

Mathias: Elisabeth, we didn't use a condom last time we had sex, so why do we have to use a condom this time?

Elisabeth: Now I know about HIV and STIs, and I want to protect myself.

Mathias: But you know that I don't have a disease. Look at me – do I look sick to you?

Elisabeth: No, you don't look sick. But we both could be sick and not even know it.

Mathias: Don't you trust me, Elisabeth?

Elisabeth: I do trust you, Mathias. Using condoms is about making sure we take care of ourselves.

Mathias: But condoms don't feel good.

Elisabeth: Let's just try it a few times. It will be more fun if we can both relax and enjoy sex instead of worrying about HIV, STIs or pregnancy.

Mathias: You are being crazy. You came here with me, so you must want to have sex.

Elisabeth: I do want to have sex with you, but only if we use a condom. Using condoms shows that we respect each other and ourselves.

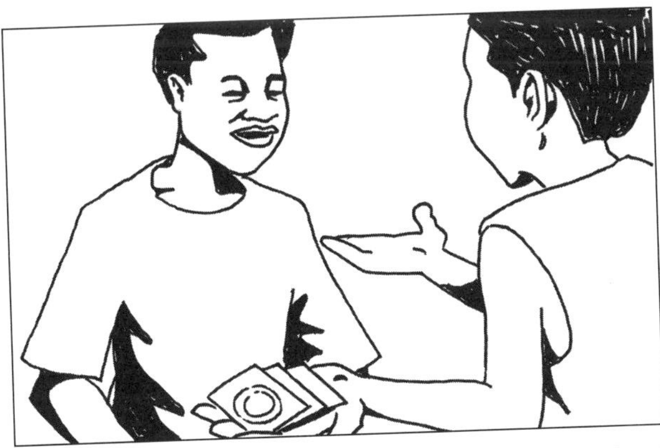

After reading Elisabeth and Mathias' story, answer the following questions:

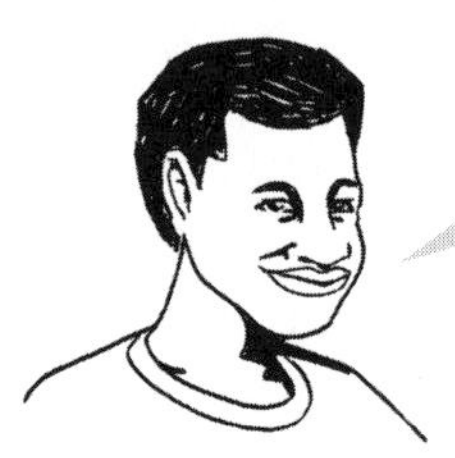

1. What do you think about Mathias and what he says?
2. What do you think about Elisabeth and what she says?
3. What would you do if you were Mathias?
4. What would you do if you were Elisabeth?
5. List reasons for using condoms for sex.

Prevention of parent to child transmission

A mother who is infected with HIV has a 1-in-3 chance of passing the virus to her child during pregnancy, labour and delivery and through breastfeeding. This is true even if the mother isn't sick with AIDS. There are ways for mothers to reduce the chances of passing the virus to their baby during pregnancy, delivery and when the mother is breastfeeding.

If a woman is pregnant, she should get tested for HIV. Knowing your HIV status is the first step to protecting your baby from becoming infected with HIV.

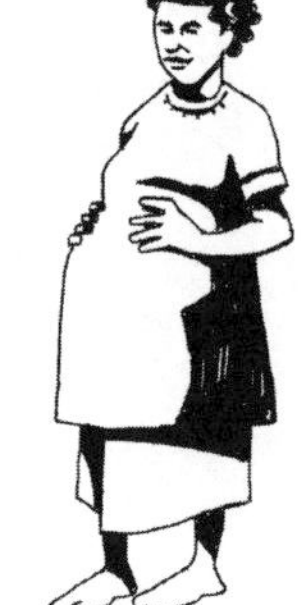

During pregnancy there are several things that HIV-infected women can do to help prevent their baby from becoming infected with HIV.

- Keep as healthy as possible by eating a healthy diet including fruit, vegetables, meat and clean water, not smoking or drinking alcohol, getting plenty of rest and getting treated for illnesses and STIs.
- Use a condom when having sex during and after pregnancy.
- Give birth by Caesarean section. A Caesarean birth is a type of surgery when a doctor makes a cut in the woman's womb and pulls the baby out. This is recommended for women infected with HIV in many countries as it reduces the chance of small tears in the baby and contact with the mother's blood. Caesarean births can only be done in a few town hospitals in PNG, so this is not an option for most pregnant women infected with HIV in PNG.
- Take antiretroviral therapy (ART). ART is only given in a few hospitals in PNG, so this is not an option for most pregnant women infected with HIV in PNG.

In Papua New Guinea, most women do not have access to a high standard of health care services in remote areas. For most women the only actions they can take to prevent their babies becoming infected with HIV is through healthy breastfeeding practices.

Breastfeeding guidelines for mothers who are infected with HIV

Breastfeeding is much safer and better for babies than bottle milk. This is because:

- in many areas of PNG the drinking water used to prepare baby formula is dirty and contaminated
- baby formula can be very expensive
- breast milk is very healthy for babies and is a good way to make sure that babies get the nutrition they need to grow properly and to stay healthy.

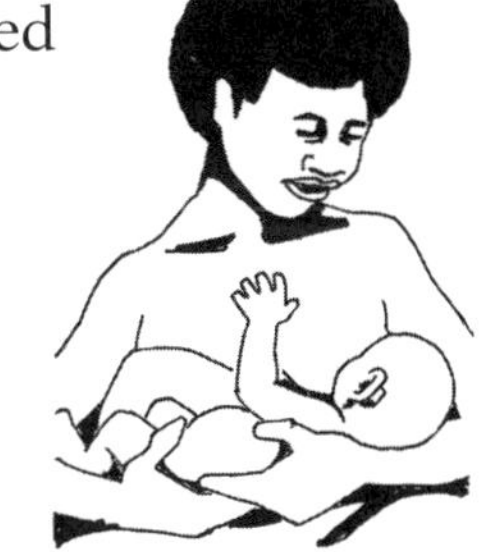

The PNG National AIDS Council recommends the following guidelines for mothers infected with HIV:

- Exclusive breastfeeding until the baby is four months old. Exclusive breastfeeding means that the baby has only breast milk – no water, no formula, no tea, no fruit or fruit juices, no honey, no sugar, no rice or dummies. These can damage the inside of the baby's mouth and stomach and make it easier for HIV to get into the baby's blood.
- When the baby is four months old the mother should stop breastfeeding and the baby should be fed other foods and liquids. Once the mother starts feeding her baby other foods, she cannot continue breastfeeding.
- Other mothers should not breastfeed the baby.

Pregnant mothers should always see a health worker.

All of our communities must look after pregnant mothers, whether they are HIV–positive or not.

 Other prevention measures

Make sure that needles for injections have been cleaned and sterilised properly or are brand new.

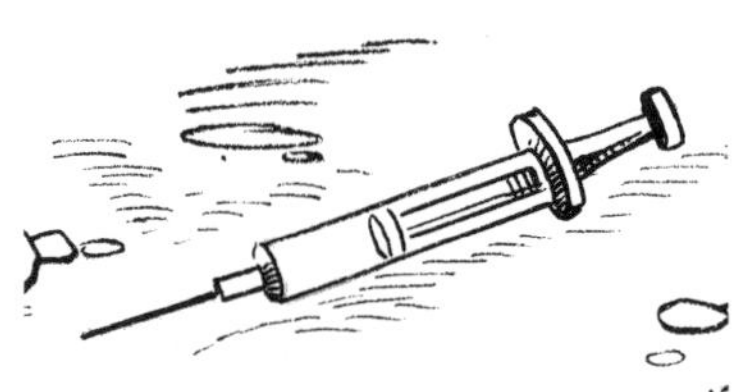

Do not share knives or blades for scarring or tattooing unless they are cleaned with strong bleach. Boiling knives and blades in water for 20 minutes will also clean and sterilise them.

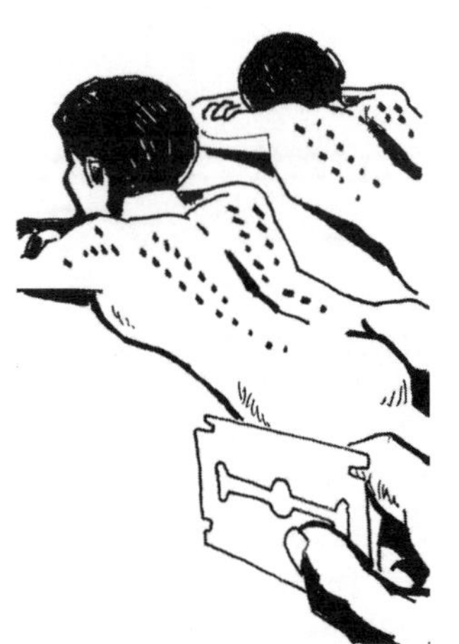

Blood spills and first aid safety – HIV cannot pass through unbroken skin, so it is safe to clean up blood and deal with injuries if there is an accident at school, in the village or while playing sport.

If you have cuts or sores on your hands, you should wear gloves to protect yourself.

Blood spills can be cleaned up with strong bleach and sand. It is best to treat all wet blood as having a potential risk and to protect yourself by wearing gloves and using bleach and clean bandages.

For more information about first aid, contact your health centre or an NGO such as the Red Cross.

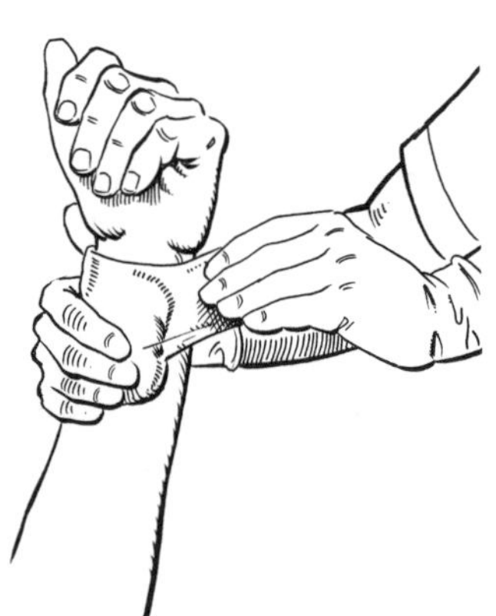

Circumcision – If a man has all of his foreskin removed, he is less likely to become infected with HIV. He should still wear a condom for sex as there is still serious risk of becoming infected with HIV or STIs. If a man has his foreskin removed and he is infected with HIV he can still pass the virus on to his sexual partners.

Strong marriage and relationships – Married couples and people in relationships can also be at risk for becoming infected with HIV and STIs. Many married people have sex with people outside of their marriage and do not always use condoms. This puts them and their partners at risk of becoming infected with HIV and STIs.

Married couples and people in relationships can use the following strategies to protect themselves and their partners from becoming infected with HIV and STIs.

- Choose your husband/wife wisely – someone who is similar in age, who has similar interests and values and who you love and care for.
- Treat your husband/wife as your equal. Treat them the way you would like to be treated.
- Work with your husband/wife to have a strong, faithful and loving relationship.
- Talk openly about your past sexual activities and other activities that may have put either of you at risk of becoming infected with HIV.
- Talk openly about using condoms to protect yourself and your partner from HIV, STIs and unwanted pregnancy.
- Talk openly about other sexual activities that will protect yourself and your partner from HIV, STIs and unwanted pregnancy.
- Get an HIV blood test to learn your HIV status and to protect your husband/wife.
- Get tested for STIs, and if necessary get treated for STIs to protect your husband/wife.

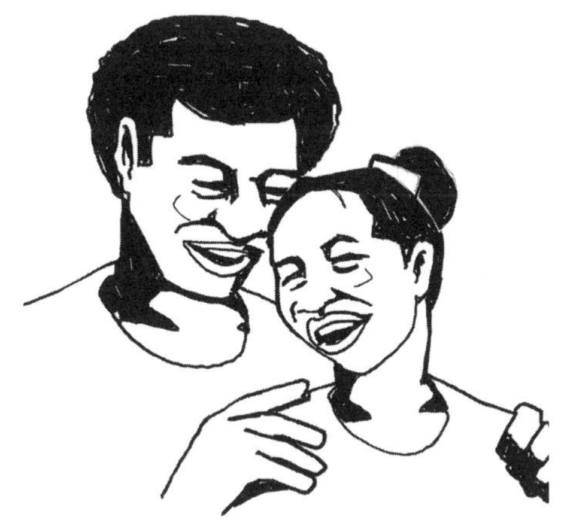

Chapter 6 Getting tested: Voluntary counselling and testing

What is VCT?

VCT stands for voluntary counselling and testing.

- **Voluntary** – This means that the person being tested has made their own decision and has not been forced by someone else to get the test.
- **Counselling** – This means that the person being tested receives counselling before and after the HIV test by a trained counsellor.
- **Testing** – This means a person will have an HIV blood test.

The only way to know if you are infected with HIV is to have an HIV blood test.

There are two types of tests for HIV in PNG. Both tests require a health worker to take a small sample of your blood.

The two kinds of tests are:

- **Rapid test:** For this test, a health worker takes a few drops of blood from the tip of the finger and puts it on a test strip. The results for this test will take 15–20 minutes. The test will show either a 'reactive' or 'negative' result. If a test is reactive, the health worker will take another blood sample and send it to a hospital lab for a confirmatory HIV-antibody test. This will make sure that the rapid test result is accurate.
- **Confirmatory HIV-antibody test:** For this test, a health worker takes blood with a needle and sends it to a hospital lab. The results for this test will take 5–10 days.

What happens when you get tested for HIV?

Making the decision to get tested for HIV

First you have to make the decision to get tested for HIV – you need the courage to go and get tested. *This decision takes place outside of the clinic.*

PNG law says that testing for HIV can only be done with a person's agreement. **This means that a person cannot be forced to have an HIV test if they do not want to have one.**

Pre-test counselling

A counsellor at the VCT centre will talk with you about HIV and the test, including:

- What is HIV?
- How is HIV transmitted?
- How is HIV prevented?
- What are risky sexual behaviours?
- What is the blood test?
- What will happen if it is positive or negative?
- What is the 'window period'?

This is an important step and you will be given as much time as you need. You can ask questions.

HIV test

The health worker will conduct the HIV test. This can be a rapid test or a confirmatory HIV-antibody test. The kind of test you take will depend on the kind of test available at the VCT centre that you visit.

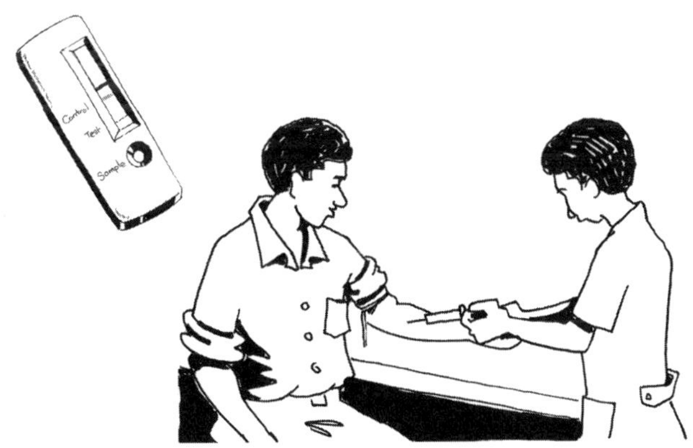

Post-test counselling

If the result is negative: You and the counsellor will discuss ways to change risky sexual behaviour in future. You might need to come back for a second HIV test in three months because of the window period.

If the result is positive before and after the confirmatory test: Counselling and support begins. You must realise that your life may be shorter but you have the power to fight the virus through **positive living** and ART. If you give up, the virus will win quickly. If you choose to fight, there are many people who can help you and your family.

It is the responsibility of the person infected with HIV to tell all their sexual partners and to encourage them to get tested for HIV.

The window period

A very important point to understand about HIV testing is that both tests look for the HIV-antibody.

- The HIV-antibody is produced by the body's immune system only when HIV has entered and infected the body.
- The body may take weeks or months after HIV infection to produce enough HIV-antibodies to be detected by an HIV test. This is called the **window period**.
- When people infected with HIV have an HIV test during the window period they will have a negative result.
- When people infected with HIV have an HIV test after the window period they will have a positive result.
- **The window period is three months.**

This means that if you have had unsafe sex in the last three months you may be in the window period. If you take an HIV test during this time you may get a negative test result but this may not be accurate. If you are infected, you can pass HIV on to your partners. To be absolutely certain about your HIV status, you should be re-tested after three months to confirm your result.

Three-month window period after having unsafe sex Even if you are HIV-positive, the test result could be negative. You should be tested again after three months.	After the three-month window period, if you are HIV positive, the HIV test result will be positive.

Unsafe sex > 1 month > 2 months > 3 months > 4 months > 5 months > 6 months

Why should I get tested for HIV?

You should get tested to find out your HIV status. You should consider getting tested if you or your partner(s) have ever:

- had vaginal or anal sex without a condom
- had sex while drunk or on drugs – you might not have used a condom
- shared needles
- shared razors or other cutting tools for tattooing, scarring or piercing.

If you are infected with HIV you can:

- get early treatment and support so you can stay healthy
- get treatment to reduce the chances of your baby getting HIV if you are pregnant
- take precautions (like using a condom) so you don't pass HIV to others.

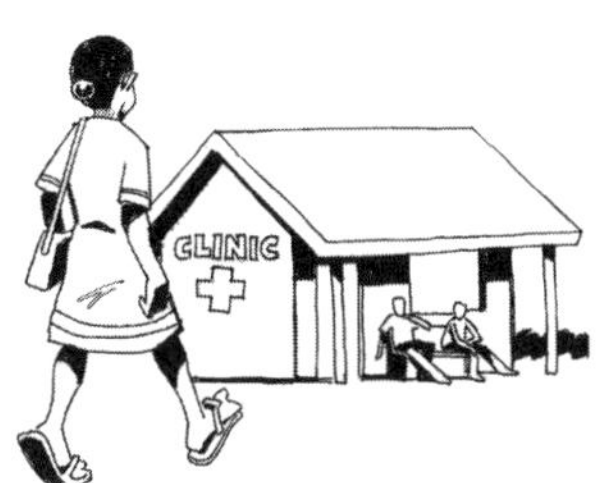

If you know that you are HIV-negative, you will have the chance to change your behaviour to avoid becoming infected with HIV. This means using condoms every time you have sex.

The information you learn through VCT gives you the power to change your life, your attitude and your sexual behaviour.

Activity 6.1 *HIV testing in your community*

Think about the following questions on HIV testing. Discuss your answers with your friends.

1. Where can you get tested for HIV in your community?
2. Why is it important to get tested for HIV?
3. Design an advertisement or poster to encourage young people to get tested for HIV.

Chapter 7 Stigma and discrimination: The HAMP Act

 Stigma and discrimination

People living with HIV often suffer from how they are treated by their family, friends and community, as well as the disease. In PNG very few people are brave enough to be public about being infected with HIV because of **stigma and discrimination**.

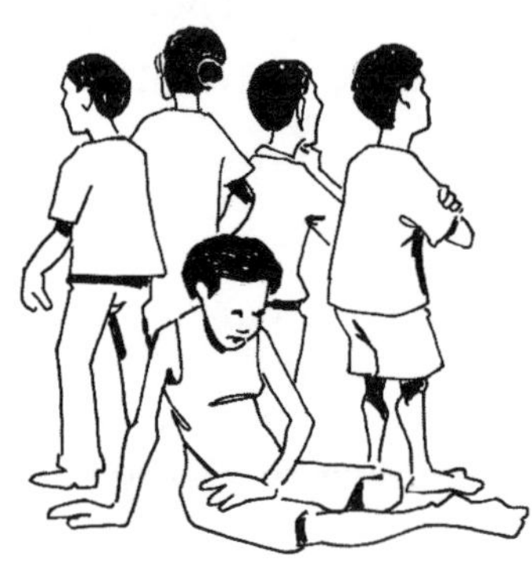

Stigma and discrimination can affect an HIV-infected person's access to treatment, employment opportunities, housing, education and other services. This kind of treatment stops people from being open about their HIV status and can lead to infection of more people.

It is against the law to treat a person living with or affected by HIV differently from other people in a way that disadvantages or harms them. This is called **discrimination**.

It is against the law to **stigmatise** people living with or affected by HIV. This means you cannot say something in public that encourages other people to hate or fear people living with or affected by HIV.

 The HAMP Act (HIV & AIDS Management and Prevention Act)

The HAMP Act was made into a law in June 2003. The HAMP Act is based on human rights. The HAMP Act recognises that abuse of people living with HIV and AIDS makes people afraid to talk about HIV and AIDS, afraid to get tested for HIV, afraid to learn about HIV and AIDS, and afraid to learn how to protect themselves and their families from becoming infected with HIV.

The HAMP Act encourages voluntary counselling and testing (VCT).

The HAMP Act states that:

- the law must protect all people whether they have HIV and AIDS or not
- all people infected with or affected by HIV should have the same rights as everyone else
- people infected with the virus should act responsibly to make sure they do not pass HIV on to anyone else.

Activity 7·2 *The stigmatised and the stigmatiser*

Sit alone quietly at a distance from other people. Think of a time in your life when you felt alone or rejected for seeming to be different from others.

1 What happened?
2 How did it feel to be treated this way?
3 What was the impact of this experience on you?

Share your stories with your classmates and community.

Next, think of a time when you rejected another person for being different.

1 What happened?
2 How did it feel to treat someone this way?
3 What was your attitude toward the person?
4 How did you behave?

Share your stories with your classmates and community.

Everybody has felt rejected or been treated poorly at some point in their lives. The thoughts, feelings and words are similar to what HIV-infected people may experience with their families and communities after telling them about their HIV status.

Many people living with HIV are rejected by their families, friends and communities, or experience other types of stigma and discrimination. Rejection and poor treatment by others can harm a person with HIV.

Stigma and discrimination go against the Melanesian and Christian values that PNG culture and society are based on.

Chapter 8 Positive living and caring for someone living with HIV

People infected with HIV can live for many years without developing AIDS. They can work, raise their children, garden, help others, play sports, and go to church – everything they would normally do.

Living positively works. People with HIV who take care of themselves and have a positive outlook on life can live much longer than other people with the virus – even without medicines or other treatments.

There are many things that people living with HIV can do to stay healthy and they should be encouraged and supported to help themselves for as long as it is possible to do so.

Activity 8.1 Positive living

- With a friend, brainstorm as many ways of keeping healthy as you can.
- Compare them to the list below.

Some things that a person living with HIV can do to live positively include:

- Do not give up on things you enjoy. Do not give up your dreams. Make plans. Keep working and stay active.
- Find people to talk to for emotional support. Tell people who are important to you that you have the virus. This may be difficult but you need their love and support.

- Avoid tobacco, drugs and alcohol. These weaken the immune system.
- Continue to look after yourself. Wash, brush your hair and teeth, change your clothes and bedding.
- Get enough rest. Always try to get a good night's sleep. Rest if you are feeling weak or tired.
- Avoid other infections. Stay away from people who are sick and try to eat clean food and drink clean water. If you get sick, go to a health worker straight away.
- Learn as much as you can about HIV and AIDS. You may need HIV medicines called ART.

People living with HIV also have a responsibility to protect others. They must tell their sexual partners that they are infected with HIV and **always** use a condom for sex. People living with HIV should avoid scar cutting and tattooing and should tell their health worker.

Caring for someone living with HIV

Caring for people living with HIV and AIDS is a responsibility we must not ignore. The current number of people living with HIV and AIDS is already putting pressure on our health services, families, communities and resources. If the number of HIV infections continues to increase, there will be serious effects to the PNG population, culture, development and economy.

People who are infected with HIV are like any other sick people but need extra care because they can get infections very easily. **People should not be afraid of people living with HIV and AIDS.**

Once AIDS has been diagnosed in a person infected with HIV, their ability to stay healthy, have a positive outlook and a good quality of life depends on the attitude and behaviour of the whole community. This includes immediate family, wantoks, friends, community leaders, employers, church leaders and health care workers. Remember, AIDS is when a person's immune system is failing.

Home-based care has many benefits. Home-based care:

- allows people to care for a person living with HIV in their communities and homes
- allows sick people to stay active in their families, communities and churches
- allows sick people to make decisions about their care
- helps sick people, their families and communities prepare for death
- helps to reduce stress or depression for people living with HIV because they are surrounded by family and friends
- provides opportunities for HIV awareness and prevention education
- contributes to reducing stigma and discrimination.

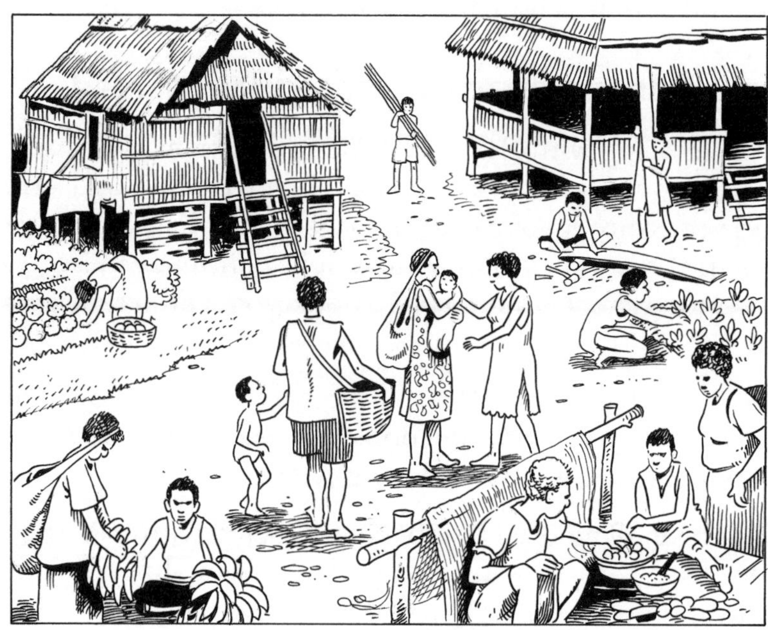

When a person is infected with HIV, their immune system is no longer able to fight off common infections. Preventing infection and sickness is the best way to protect a person living with HIV and to help them live a longer life. It is also important to treat infections when they occur, to help the person stay healthy for as long as possible. Caring for someone living with HIV and AIDS can be stressful and tiring. People living with AIDS need a lot of care, especially near the end of their lives.

Some things that can be done to care for a person living with HIV include:

1. Wash your hands with soap and water:
   - before and after caring for them
   - after using the toilet or changing diapers
   - after changing bedding
   - before cooking, eating, or feeding another person.

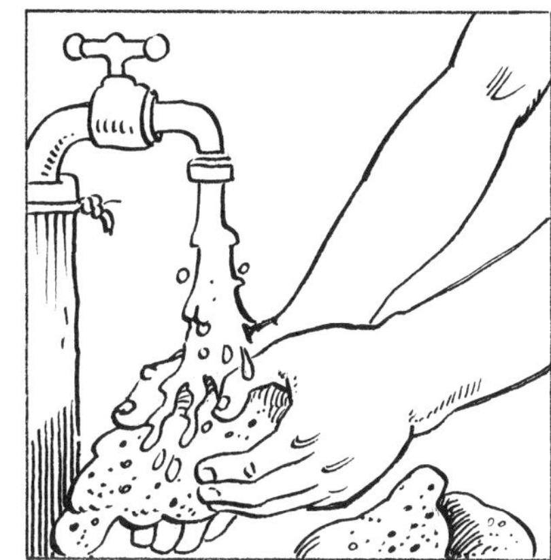

2. Keep food safe:
   - Always use clean, boiled water for drinking and cooking.
   - Eggs, meat and shellfish should be well cooked.
   - Wash fruits and vegetables in clean water.
   - Store all food and water in a clean, cool place and keep containers covered.
   - Protect food from insects, rats and other animals.
   - Clean the cooking area and utensils with soap and clean water.

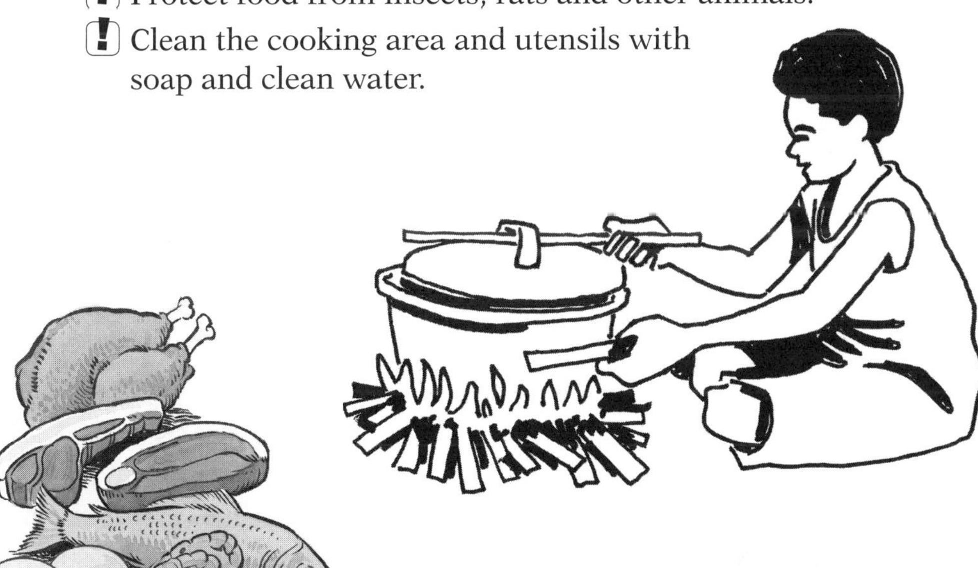

3. Wash and bleach dirty clothes and bedding to make sure the person living with HIV has less chance of catching other germs. (Use one part bleach to six parts water and soak for 20 minutes.)

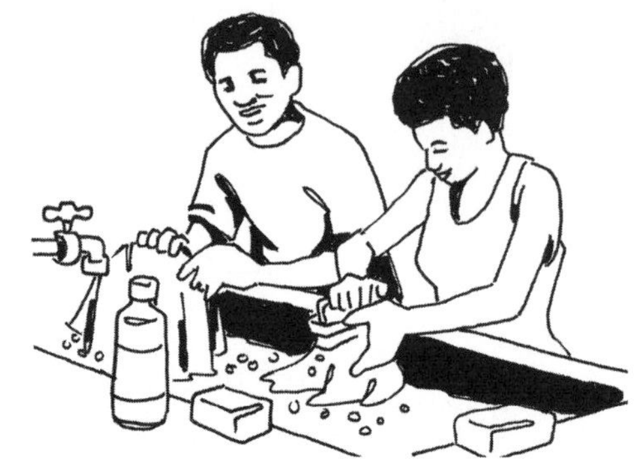

4. Wash razors and toothbrushes in soapy water or a very weak mix of bleach and water.
5. Do not share anything that touches blood, such as needles, razors or cutting tools used for tattoos or skin piercing.
6. Get a health worker if the person develops a cough (it could be TB), has diarrhoea or vomits. They should take medicine for other infections.
7. Get a health worker if the person living with HIV is in too much pain or has an infection that will not heal.
8. Help the person living with HIV to take ART and other medicines properly and according to the health care worker's instructions.

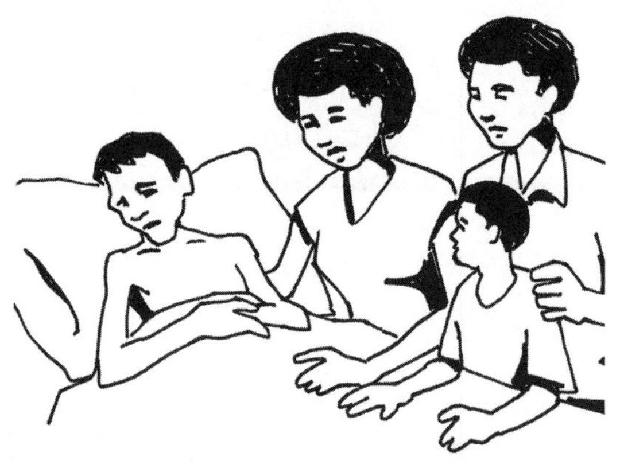

9. Help the person living with HIV to prepare for the future and the life of their family after they have died.
10. Don't forget to look after the caregiver. Caring for a person living with HIV takes a lot of time and energy. Caregivers must get enough rest and food and make sure that they look after their own health and wellbeing. Try to organise a group of people from the community to take turns looking after the person living with HIV.
11. Ask for help if you need it or if you are upset. Many churches and NGOs offer support with home care.

Activity 8.2 *Support for people affected by HIV*

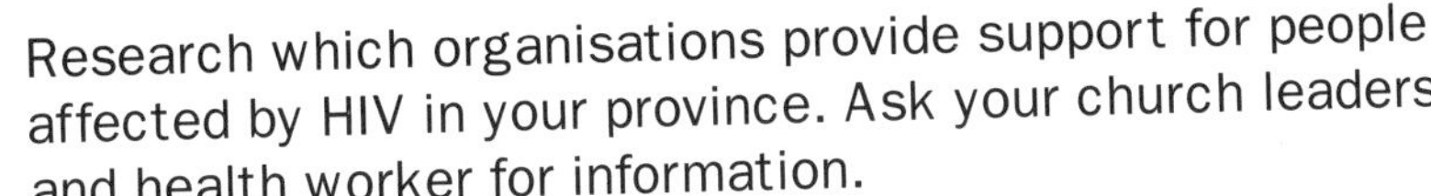

Research which organisations provide support for people affected by HIV in your province. Ask your church leaders and health worker for information.

Home care supply kits

If you are caring for someone who is living with AIDS you will need a home care supply kit containing household equipment such as buckets, dishes and a secure dry box or other container for medicines.

All medicines should be kept in a safe, cool, dry place away from children and animals. The sick person will also need basic medical supplies. The caregiver should contact the nearest health service provider so that the person living with HIV and AIDS can receive necessary medicines.

If you require help, the following organisations may be able to assist you:

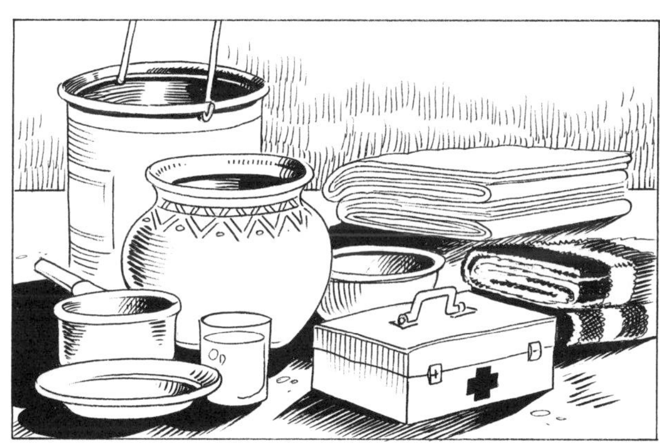

- provincial AIDS committee
- local health care provider
- hospital
- NGO
- church.

Do not be afraid. Do not let people spread nasty stories or false information – tell them the facts about HIV.

Get help from your local health worker for support and to educate your neighbours, family and friends about HIV and AIDS.

Treatment for people living with HIV

There is no cure for HIV or AIDS.

Treatment for symptoms and opportunistic infections

Good home-based care can do a lot to lessen the symptoms of opportunistic infections such as vomiting, diarrhoea, fever, sweating, itching, pain and breathing problems. Treatment of opportunistic infections can also help a person living with HIV live a longer and more productive life.

Basic medicines such as Panadol, antiseptic cream and oral rehydration solutions are useful. It is important to take antibiotics given by health care providers properly and completely according to the health care worker's instructions.

Tuberculosis (TB) is one of the most common opportunistic infections for people living with HIV, so it is important to treat TB. If a person living with HIV has a cough, they should see a health worker immediately.

Traditional medicines

Be aware of false information!

Local homemade herbal remedies and traditional healers can be helpful to lessen the symptoms of opportunistic infections. Any remedy that can bring peace of mind and doesn't cause any other health problems may contribute to better health for someone living with HIV.

There are people in PNG who try to make people believe that they have special medicines and cures for HIV and AIDS. These people are only trying to take your money and take advantage of you. Do not waste your money.

None of these medicines can cure HIV.

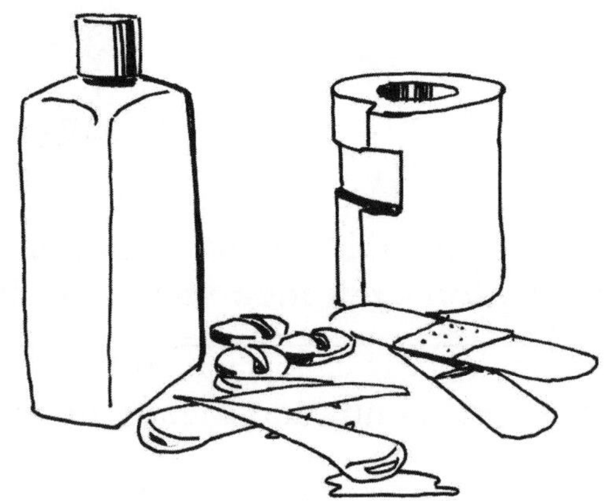

Antiretroviral therapies (ARTs)

The medicines used to treat HIV infections are called antiretroviral therapies (ARTs).

ARTs prevent HIV from multiplying in the body. These drugs do not remove the virus from the body or cure HIV. They work by slowing down the body's production of HIV. ARTs help to reduce the level of HIV in the blood, to make the immune system stronger and to keep people healthy longer.

Even though ARTs are better than any other treatment, there are some problems:

- ART can have very bad side-effects like nausea, dizziness, headaches and high blood pressure. Many people have had to stop treatment due to very bad side-effects.
- ART is provided free in PNG, but many people cannot afford to travel regularly to health centres and hospitals that provide these medicines.
- ART requires people to take many pills each day for the rest of their lives.
- Researchers do not know the long-term effects of these medicines or how well they work over time.

Activity 8.3 *Caring for someone living with HIV*

- Prepare a drama with your friends that shows the Melanesian and Christian ways of caring for someone who is sick with AIDS.
- Perform your drama for your friends and family.

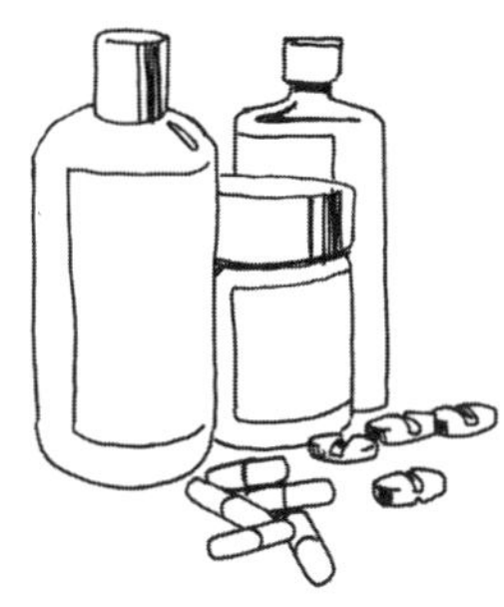

Chapter 9 HIV and AIDS and their future impact on PNG

HIV and AIDS are damaging the future of PNG. Men and women contribute in many ways to PNG culture, development and economy and many of these people are becoming infected with HIV and dying from AIDS. These people are community leaders, politicians, doctors, teachers, parents, children and many, many more.

We need to protect these people and prevent them from becoming infected with HIV. They are the future of PNG.

The table below predicts what the HIV situation might look like in PNG in 2010, 2015 and 2025.

Predicted number of people living with HIV in PNG (2005, 2010, 2015, 2025)

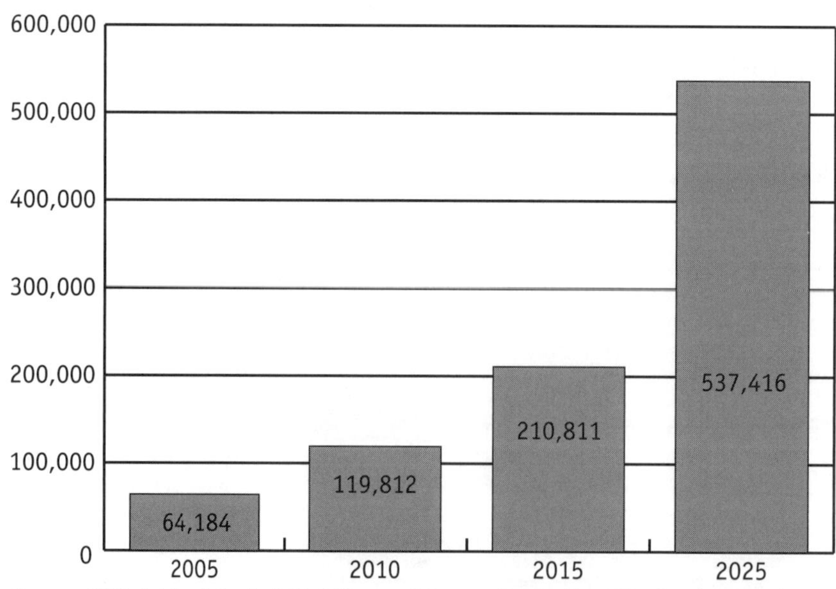

Source: HIV Epidemiological Modelling and Impact Study (AusAID, October 2005)

According to this table, by 2025:

- there will be more than 500 000 people living with HIV in PNG
- more than 10% of adults will be infected with HIV
- 300 000 adults will have died due to HIV-related illnesses
- 117 000 children will lose their mother to HIV.

This will have great effects on PNG.

- It will affect social welfare, the economy, the government and health and education services.
- This will be a great threat to culture, health and economic and social development.
- The cost of treating HIV and AIDS will cause a big strain on families, communities, government services and all other sectors of society.
- The cost of health services will increase and resources will be taken from other services to pay for these costs.

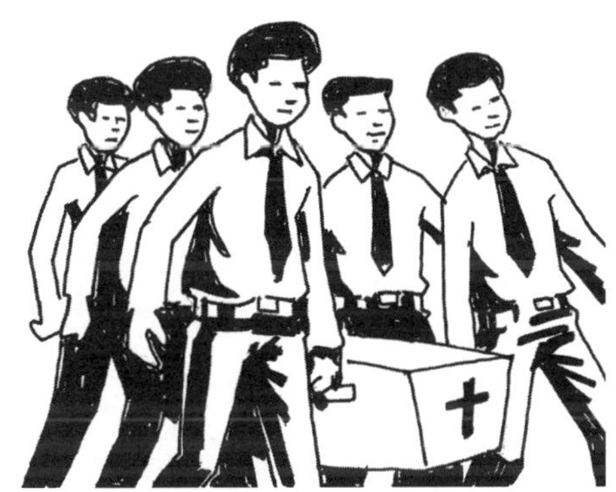

This situation can be prevented if:

- people change their behaviours (use condoms, have fewer sexual partners, are faithful to their partners and start having sex at an older age)
- leaders take action in their response
- health services are improved, strengthened and supported
- the number of awareness programs and support services increases
- people get tested for HIV and know their status
- people start talking openly about HIV and AIDS.

Activity 9.1 *HIV in my community*

Think about the effects of the HIV epidemic on your community in the future and answer the questions below. Discuss your answers with friends and family.

1. What can young people do to prevent HIV from seriously affecting their communities?
2. Imagine your community in 2025. If the HIV epidemic is not controlled, what will your community be like?
3. What will you do to prevent HIV? Write an action plan for yourself.

AIDS IS EVERYONE'S PROBLEM!
A PERSON WITH AIDS IS JUST LIKE YOU AND ME

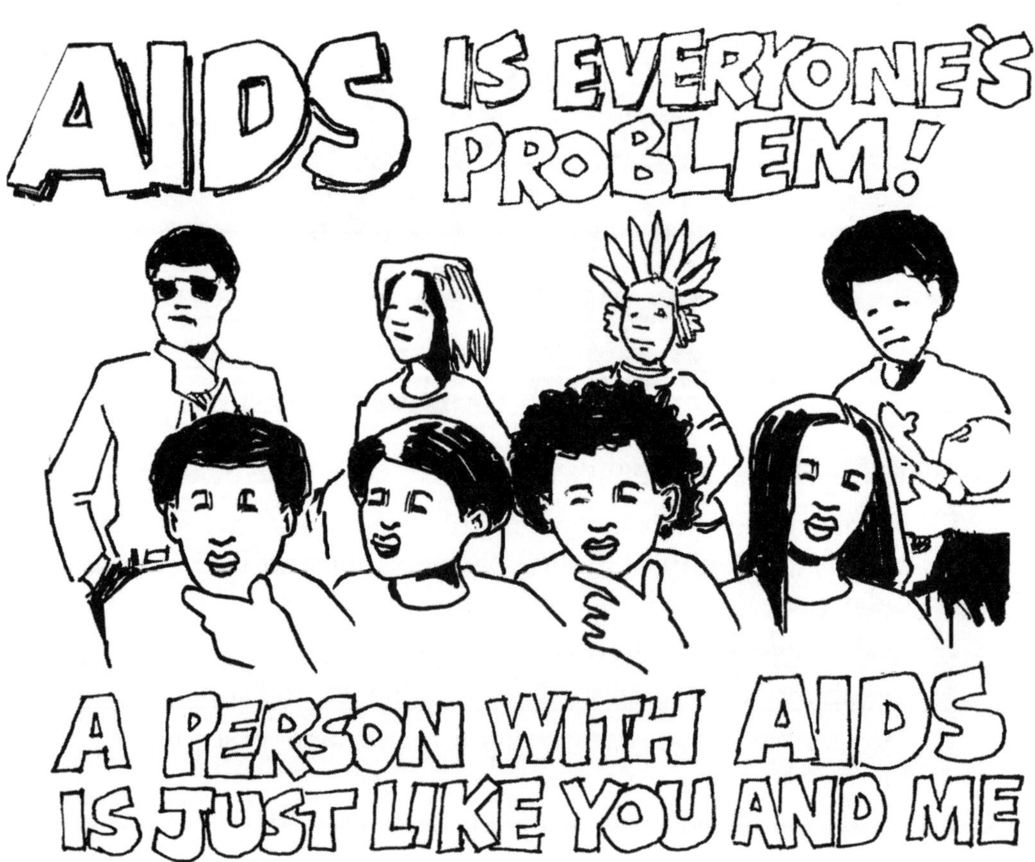

Chapter 10 Sexually transmitted infections in PNG

PNG has the highest rate of STI infection in the Pacific. The most common STIs in PNG are gonorrhoea, chlamydia, donovanosis, syphilis, thrush, herpes and HIV. The table beginning on page 56 outlines the symptoms, treatment and medical problems caused by these infections.

Because there are many different STIs, there are many different symptoms. Some STIs don't have any symptoms at all.

Common symptoms in women include:

- discharge from the vagina that is thick, itchy, or has an unusual smell or colour
- pain in the lower stomach area
- pain or burning feeling when passing urine (peeing)
- pain during sex
- irregular bleeding from the vagina
- itching in the genital area
- swelling or growths in the genital area
- sores, blisters, ulcers, warts or rashes around the genital area.

Common symptoms in men include:

- a wound, sore, ulcer, rash, or blister on or around the penis
- a discharge, like pus, from the penis
- pain or burning feeling when passing urine (peeing)
- pain during sex
- pain and swelling of the testicles
- swelling or growths in the genital area
- sores, blisters, ulcers, warts or rashes around the genital area.

Often STIs do not have symptoms. Sometimes there are symptoms at the start of infection and then the symptoms go away. This does not mean that the infection has gone away. You will still have the infection and it will be doing damage to your body.

Prevention of STIs

STIs are transmitted through unprotected sexual activities. The best ways to prevent STIs are the same as the prevention measures for HIV:

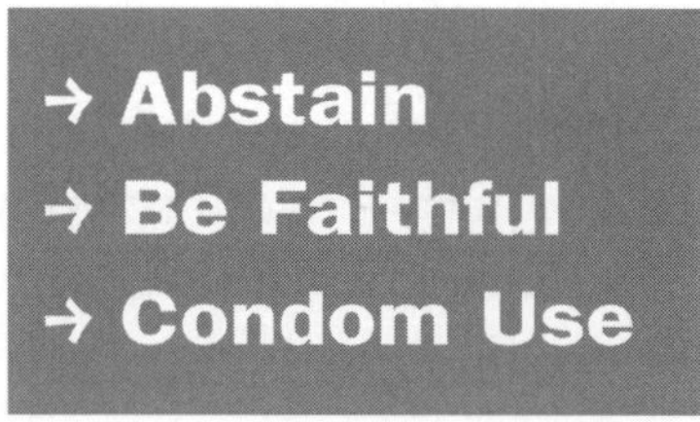

Having safe sex and using a condom makes you much less likely to get an STI.

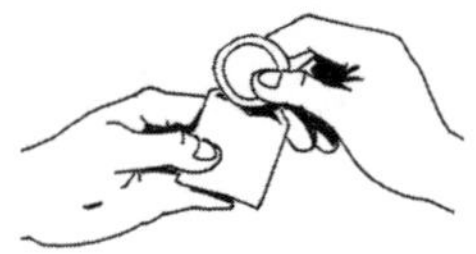

Treatment for STIs

If your body shows any of the symptoms listed above or if you have had unsafe sex, you may have become infected with an STI. You should visit a doctor or health clinic as soon as possible to prevent the infection from developing further.

Many STIs can be easily detected, treated and cured. If you think that you have an STI, you and your partner should get treatment as soon as possible. Many people ignore early symptoms until more serious damage is done. If untreated, STIs can lead to serious long-term health problems and permanent damage to your reproductive system. People with an untreated STI can infect their partner(s) with STIs.

STIs and HIV

All STIs, especially those that cause sores, make it easier for HIV to be transmitted from one person to another. This is because:

- STIs that cause sores, blisters or discharge make it easier for HIV to get into the blood. These sores act as a 'doorway' for HIV to pass into the body
- HIV infects white blood cells, and there are a high number of white blood cells found at the site of an STI infection
- the discharge associated with some STIs contains a lot of HIV
- HIV damages the immune system and makes it easier for the body to become infected with other infections, including STIs
- getting an STI is a sign that you have had unprotected sex and your partner may also have had unprotected sex with someone else.

If you think you have an STI you must get treated. Your sexual partner must also be tested and treated.

If you have an STI you and your partner must change your sexual behaviour.

Table of STIs, symptoms and treatment

Infection	Symptoms in women	Symptoms in men	Treatment	Medical problems if STI is not treated
Chlamydia (bacteria)	Usually no symptoms – increased vaginal discharge or irritation during urination, irregular bleeding	Usually no symptoms – sometimes pain during urination and discharge from penis. Can cause heaviness and inflammation of the testicles and a small, hard area of painful swelling at the base of the testicles.	• Cured with antibiotics	• Infertility • Eye damage in babies if woman giving birth has chlamydia
Donovanosis (bacteria)	Small red bumps on the penis or vagina and around the anus which bleed easily. The sores might be painless. Eventually these can become large ulcers.		• Cured with antibiotics	• Ulcers will become larger and parts of the genitals will be destroyed • Infection may spread to other parts of the body
Genital herpes (virus)	Discomfort or itching with small blisters appearing in infected areas of the skin, usually the genital area. Fever can occur. After a few days, blisters form a thin yellowish crust which disappears in 10–12 days. Blisters can recur.		• Symptoms can be treated with drugs, but the virus remains in the body and the infection cannot be cured	• Urinary problems, possible meningitis in the most severe cases • Increases risk of cancer

Infection	Symptoms in women	Symptoms in men	Treatment	Medical problems if STI is not treated
Genital warts (Human Papilloma Virus)	Tiny painless lumps (cauliflower-like) around vagina, penis or anus. Sometimes no symptoms.		• Treated with freezing or special paint • Virus remains in the body and can reappear later	• Linked to cervical cancer
Gonorrhoea (bacteria)	Pain when urinating	Heaviness, pain and inflammation of the testicles Heavy pus-like discharge and pain when urinating	• Cured with antibiotics	• Infertility • Blindness in babies if woman giving birth has gonorrhoea • Painful swelling of joints • Damage to heart and liver
	Many people have gonorrhoea but have no symptoms at all. A person without any symptoms can still pass the infection on and may develop complications from the infection.			
HIV (Human Immunodeficiency Virus)	Infected people show no symptoms for many years (may have flu-like symptoms shortly after infection). Lifelong damage to immune system and AIDS conditions begin between 1 and 20 years after infection.		• No vaccine or cure. Antiretroviral therapy keeps people healthier for longer	• AIDS-related illnesses such as TB, pneumonia and diarrhoea

Infection	Symptoms in women	Symptoms in men	Treatment	Medical problems if STI is not treated
Syphilis (bacteria)	**Primary syphilis:** A small pimple appears where the bacteria entered the body, usually on the penis or inside of the vagina. A colourless, infectious liquid oozes from the pimple. The sore disappears by itself without medication, but the bacteria will spread to other parts of the body. **Secondary syphilis:** A few weeks or months after the sore disappears the following symptoms may appear: • Fever • Swelling in the groin, armpits and neck • Sores appear in the moist parts of the body (mouth, genitals and armpits) • Skin develops a dry, scaly rash These symptoms disappear within a couple of weeks if left untreated, but the bacteria are still in the body. **Tertiary syphilis:** The infection continues to attack the body and may affect organs such as the heart, brain and bones.		• Cured with antibiotics	• If left untreated, syphilis may result in blindness, heart trouble, poor mental health and death
Thrush (candida) (fungus)	Creamy thick discharge, smelly, itchy and inflamed vagina. Can also be caused by stress or use of antibiotics.	Itchy rash on penis or anus. Can be found in mouth and throat.	• Antifungal creams and other natural options	

What have we learnt?

- Having any kind of unprotected sex can put people at risk of becoming infected with STIs and HIV.
- HIV is a virus that weakens the body's immune system so that it is no longer able to protect itself from infections.
- AIDS refers to the group of opportunistic infections (illnesses) that a person who is infected with HIV becomes sick with when their immune system is weakened.
- A person living with HIV can feel and look healthy for many years after he or she is infected. During this time the infected person can infect other people.
- There is no cure for HIV or AIDS.
- HIV is found in four types of body fluids: blood, semen, vaginal fluids and breast milk.
- HIV is passed from one person to another through unprotected sex, blood-to-blood contact and parent to child transmission.
- People can protect themselves from becoming infected with HIV and other STIs by abstaining from sex, being faithful to a partner who is also free of HIV, using a male or female condom during sex, and not sharing needles or other cutting instruments.
- Condoms are a proven way to prevent the spread of HIV and other STIs when they are used consistently and correctly.
- The only way to know if you are infected with HIV is to have an HIV blood test.
- Knowing your HIV status will help you to plan for the future, make more informed choices, take the steps to live a longer healthier life and protect others from becoming infected.
- Home-based care is an important way to care for people living with HIV.

- Love and support from family, friends, churches and communities can help people living with HIV to live longer, healthier lives.
- STIs are infectious diseases that are passed from one person to another through sexual contact. HIV is one of the most serious STIs.
- Common STIs in PNG are HIV, gonorrhoea, chlamydia, syphilis, thrush, herpes and donovanosis.
- STIs often have no symptoms or the symptoms take a long time to develop.
- If you have symptoms of an STI, you should go to a health centre or clinic for treatment and care

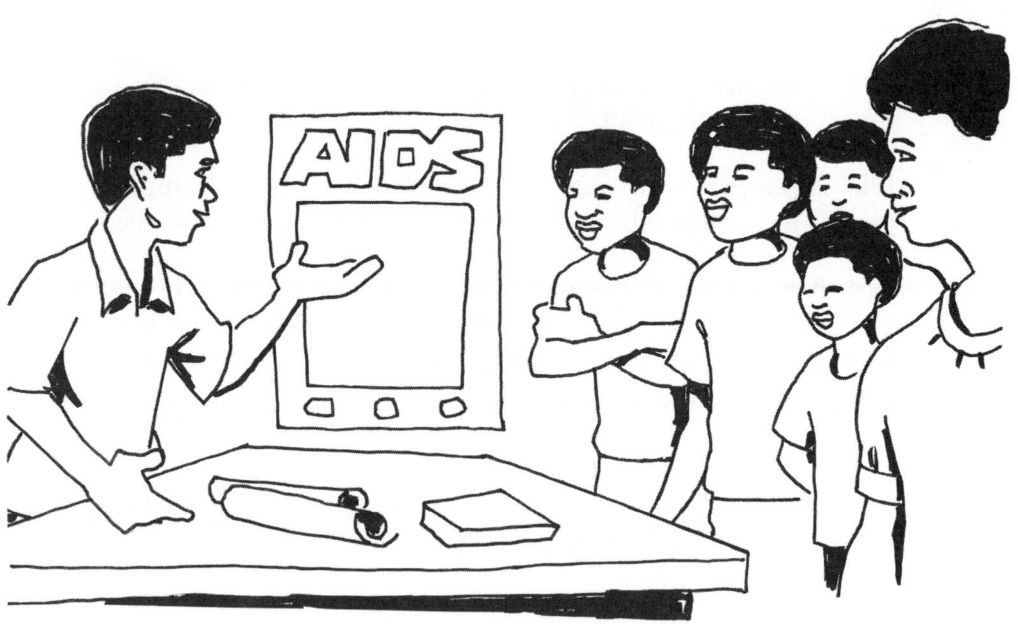

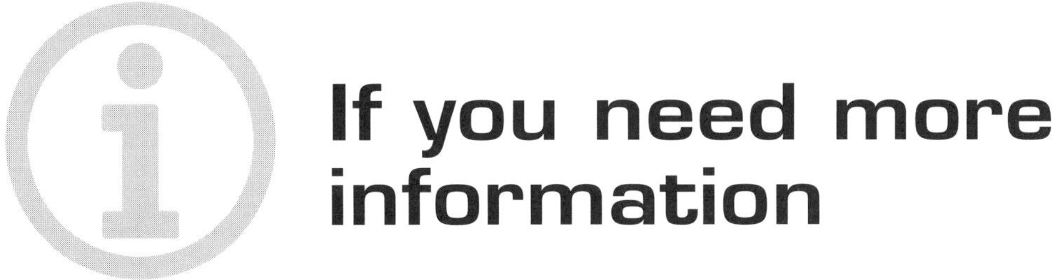

If you need more information

There are many organisations in PNG that provide HIV and AIDS and STI services. They have many resources that they can share with you. They are ready and willing to listen and help.

For more information, please contact:

National AIDS Council
323-6161
NCD
Provincial AIDS Committee

Bougainville (Buka) 973-9191
Central (Konedobu) 321-6032
East Sepik (Wewak) 856-1844
East New Britain (Rabaul) 982-9525
Eastern Highlands (Goroka) 732-2299
Enga (Wabag) 547-1141
Gulf (Kerema) 648-1285
Madang (Madang) 852-3422
Manus (Lorengau) 470-9643
Milne Bay (Alotau) 641-0433
Morobe (Lae) 472-0644
NCD (Port Moresby) 323-0166
Oro (Popondetta) 329-7782
Sandaun (Vanimo) 857-1404
Simbu (Kundiawa) 735-1203
Southern Highlands (Mendi) 549-1710
West New Britain (Kimbe) 983-5492
Western (Daru) 645-9090
Western Highlands (Mt Hagen) 542-3835

Other HIV and AIDS service providers in your area

Activity *Community mapping*

Draw a map of your community and mark the locations of churches, schools, health care providers, organisations and other important places or people in your community.

Think about all of the people and places where you can learn more about HIV, AIDS and STIs. Put these people and places on your map. Make a list of places outside of your community where you can learn more about HIV, AIDS and STIs.

Compare your community map with those of your classmates and friends.

Glossary

abstinence — choosing not to have sex (oral, anal, vaginal) at all

acquired immune deficiency syndrome (AIDS) — the group of illnesses that a person becomes sick with when they are infected with HIV. AIDS is caused by HIV, which damages the body's immune system

anal intercourse — a form of sexual intercourse where a man puts his penis inside the anus of a woman or a man

antibodies — particles produced by the body's immune system in response to an infection

circumcision — an operation when the foreskin is cut away from a boy's or a man's penis

condom — male condom refers to a rubber sheath or tube worn on a man's penis during sex to prevent pregnancy and the transmission of HIV and STIs

female condom refers to a plastic liner inserted into the woman's vagina during sex to prevent pregnancy and the transmission of HIV and STIs

gay — refers to someone who finds people of the same sex attractive and may have sex with them

gender and sex — the term 'gender' describes the roles given to women and men by the society and culture in which they live. The term 'sex' refers to biological characteristics. Using the term 'gender' highlights the fact that men and women behave differently not only because of their biological sex (what they were born with), but also because of what their society or community has taught them about how men and women are supposed to behave

germ — any micro-organism (for example, a bacterium, virus, or parasite), especially one that causes disease

human immunodeficiency virus (HIV) — the virus that weakens the immune system and leads to AIDS

heterosexual (straight) refers to someone who is attracted to and may have sex with someone of the opposite sex

HIV-infected as distinct from HIV-positive. The term HIV-infected is usually used to indicate that evidence of HIV has been found through an HIV blood test

HIV-negative showing no evidence of infection with HIV (e.g. absence of antibodies against HIV) in an HIV blood test. An HIV-negative person can be infected with HIV if he or she is in the window period between HIV exposure and detection of antibodies

HIV-positive showing indications of being infected with HIV (e.g. presence of antibodies against HIV) on a blood test. This is the same as 'seropositive'. A test may rarely show a false positive result

homosexual (gay) refers to someone who is attracted to and may have sex with someone of the same sex: men with men or women with women

immune system the body system which fights infection

infection when a micro-organism enters a person's body, making them ill. Viruses, bacteria and fungi can all cause infection in people

intercourse (sex) when a man puts his penis into a woman's vagina it is called vaginal intercourse. When a man puts his penis into a man's or woman's anus (back passage) it is called anal intercourse

opportunistic infections infections that take advantage of a person's weakened immune system to cause illness, such as TB, pneumonia and diarrhoea

oral sex when a person uses his or her mouth and tongue to lick or suck a sexual partner's genitals

penis the male sexual organ. The penis hangs between a male's legs and becomes larger and harder when it is erect

people living with HIV (PLWHIV) refers to people who are living with HIV

safe sex sex during which HIV is less likely to be spread, such as vaginal or anal sex with a condom

scarification	the cultural practice of using sharp instruments to cut a person's skin to leave a permanent scar
semen	the thick liquid that comes out from a man's penis during sex. Semen contains sperm and can carry HIV
sex worker	the term 'sex worker' is non-judgmental and recognises the fact that some people sell their bodies as a way to survive or to earn a living. This term is better than 'prostitute', 'whore' or 'commercial sex worker', which are negative
sexually transmitted infection (STI)	an infection spread from person to person through sexual contact
sterilisation	the process for cleaning needles and instruments that kills germs and prevents the spread of disease
symptom	a sign of an infection, disease or disorder
syndrome	a group of symptoms or diseases that are used to define an illness
syringe	a glass or plastic tube attached to a hollow needle used to inject medicine or take blood out of the body
unsafe sex	sex during which HIV is likely to be spread, such as vaginal or anal sex without a condom
vagina	the passage leading from the uterus to the vulva in a female. During sex, a man puts his penis inside the woman's vagina
vaginal intercourse (sex)	when a man puts his penis in a woman's vagina
virus	extremely small germs that can cause many infections
voluntary counselling and testing (VCT)	refers to the process of getting tested for HIV. This includes counselling before and after the HIV blood test by a trained health worker
window period	the time between infection with HIV and the development of antibodies to the virus (three months)

Notes

Notes